PARENTS TALK LOVE

PARENTS TALK LOVE

THE CATHOLIC FAMILY HANDBOOK ABOUT SEXUALITY

Susan K. Sullivan
Matthew A. Kawiak

Paulist Press
New York/Mahwah

Photo Credits:

Robert L. Beckhard, p. xii, 118
Tom McCarthy, p. 10
Paul S. Conklin, p. 26, 70
Rick Smolan, p. 52, 88
Kay Freeman, p. 104
Vera Wulf, p. 152
Vivienne della Grotta, cover photo

Nihil Obstat:
Rev. Msgr. William H. Shannon

Imprimatur:
Matthew H. Clark,
Bishop of Rochester

Date:
June 27, 1984

The Nihil Obstat and Imprimatur are official declarations that a book or pamphlet is free of doctrinal or moral error. No implication is contained therein that those who have granted the Nihil Obstat and Imprimatur agree with the contents, opinions or statements expressed.

Library of Congress
Catalog Card Number: 84-80361

ISBN: 0-8091-2639-7

Published by Paulist Press
997 Macarthur Boulevard
Mahwah, New Jersey 07430

Printed and bound in the
United States of America

Contents

Preface

At a parish youth workshop on sexuality, teenagers are encouraged to share the messages they most want to hear from their parents. A frequent plea from young people is for parents to listen and not lecture. One high school senior explained: "We don't need another scolding; what we really need is someone who lets us talk and is willing to listen to us." It is significant that young people want and need to discuss sexual matters with their parents. It is also significant that since Vatican II, the Catholic Church has encouraged parents especially to provide "a positive and prudent sex education" to children and young people. The most recent guidelines for sex education, entitled "Educational Guidance in Human Love" and issued in December 1983 by the Vatican Congregation for Catholic Education, stress that the family is "the best environment to accomplish the obligation of securing a gradual education in sexual life." Unfortunately, these messages are ignored, ridiculed or suppressed by people who have grown insensitive to the need for young people to be informed with the information and values our Catholic tradition has upheld as essential in the personal maturity of every person. Rather than silence, this Vatican document has chosen to challenge parents to "establish a relationship of trust and of dialogue with the children in a manner appropriate to their age and development."

Young people need to see and experience, within their own families, the free and easy expression of love and affection. They need to be listened to, to feel accepted, and to feel warmth. They need to be embraced and hugged. Children first learn about sex in their own home without words. Life in the family "talks" to them incessantly about human relationships. If parents are unashamed in their physical and verbal expression of love and affection, then children are powerfully influenced for good. The Vatican statement asserts the essential role of the family in this educational process when it states: "Christian parents must know that their example represents the most valid contribution in the education of their children.''

In our separate roles as parish priest and parochial school teacher, we have confronted the controversy and struggle of many parents who still feel embarrassed, confused, angry and ashamed when talking about masturbation, birth control and homosexuality. Our purpose in writing this book is to bring a message of comfort, a touch of confidence, and a word of encouragement to the hearts of all Catholic parents who have understood God's fascinating gift of sexuality as the Creator's communion with us. The Vatican recognizes that this task of education belongs primarily to the family, but that the family also requires the help of ''pastors . . . involved in the preparation of responsible personnel and in the determination of content and method.'' The primary message we want Catholic parents to pass on to the next generation of young people is that our sexuality has always been intended by God to be ''understood, affirmed and celebrated.''

Many parents already feel this way about sexuality in their hearts, but where did they learn it? Certainly not from the pulpit during a Sunday homily, or in the confessional on a Saturday afternoon. It was seldom taught in a classroom, and rarely was sex discussed in the home. Our discussions at workshops, conferences in the school, and counseling in the office have taught us how uncomfortable parents, quite understandably, feel in talking about sexuality with their children. Many parents, while striving to conform to the Church's sexual moral teachings, struggle with certain sexual issues and are living contrary to official Catholic teaching. As a result, parents feel helpless, for they might see themselves as poor models for their children to follow and, worse yet, decide not to provide the guidance children desperately need in dealing with the more sensitive issues. Contrary to much modern therapy, we suggest that it simply is not necessary to feel totally comfortable about your own or anybody else's sexuality in order to assume the special role of sex educator of your child. The aim of this book will be to challenge how you think and feel about being a sexual person. Our intention is to help parents create an environment which encourages open and honest communication about sexuality and enriches the relationship between parents and their children. We strongly encourage that this book be read by all manner of parents: single, married partners, adopting, foster, grandparents, mothers and especially fathers. The core of this book is an extensive selection of read-and-discuss questions designed to give parents the opportunity to prepare themselves to handle discussion of sexuality with their children; and we shall strive to deal very directly, and truthfully, with the more difficult topics such as masturbation, intercourse, contraception and venereal disease.

We understand the risks that most parents assume will come in discussing sexuality openly and honestly with their children. Yet the risks run by a conspiracy of silence can lead to far greater harm. The Vatican document identifies a fundamental need ''to protect (children and young people) from the dangers of ignorance and widespread degradation.'' Young people, swamped by the open sexuality in the media, are searching for guidance in coping with it and their own sexuality. Parents must become the primary resource for answering their questions within the context of faith, morality and religious tradition. Sexuality education must be an integral part of all Church family life education programs.

The recent magisterium's declarations on sex education strongly support "a solid catechetical preparation of adults on human love" as the foundation for dialogue with our children and young people on sexuality. It is the wish of John Paul II that parents take a more careful and honest look into the fascinating mystery of human sexuality as God created and intended. We have designed *Parents Talk Love* to become part of a much needed healing ministry in our Catholic Church, to remove the pain of irrational and unnecessary guilt from an area of life God designed to be a refuge from loneliness and reserved for intimate sharing. The *Declaration on Christian Education* of Vatican II affirmed the right of young people to receive an education adequate to their personal requirements. Furthermore, the Pope's encyclical on the mission of the Christian family emphasizes: "Education to love as self-giving constitutes the indispensable premise for parents called to offer their children a clear and delicate sex education." The Catholic Church has a definite mandate to teach sexuality within the context of our faith and moral tradition. *Parents Talk Love* will underline and focus on the many positive, life-affirming and compassionate messages held by our tradition. As you go through this guide, the difficulties encountered in teaching sexuality to children will never disappear, but instead of crushing us, they will become stepping stones to family holiness today and for many generations to come.

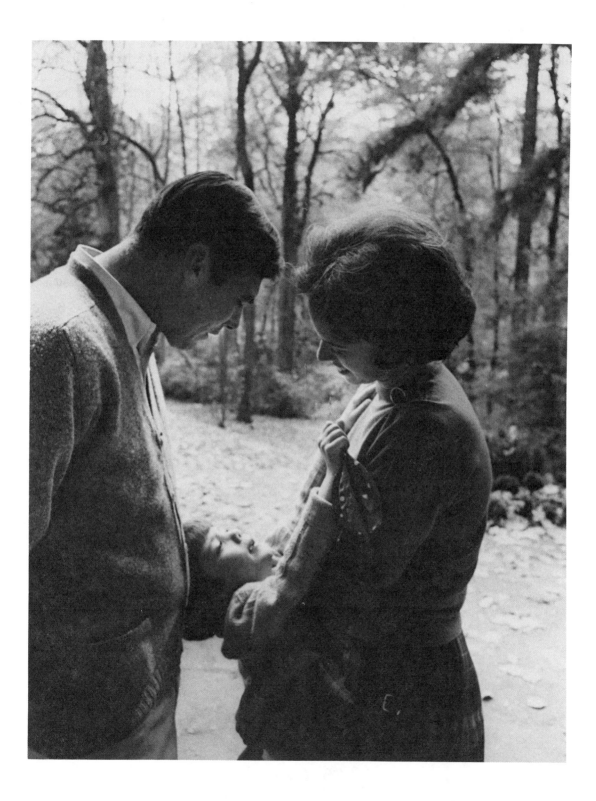

Sexuality Education—
A Parental Responsibility

Not too long ago in a suburban parochial school, a disturbing thing happened. A frantic mother phoned to talk about her fifth grade daughter. It seems the girl had been acting unusual, asking her sisters if they thought she was putting on weight. She had trouble sleeping at night. She felt moody and not her usual happy-go-lucky self. This had been going on for almost two weeks before the mother finally sat down with her ten year old for a serious talk. With a good bit of coaxing, questioning, and a few tears, the whole story came out. For over two weeks the girl had lived in agony and fear, convinced that she was going to have a baby. She had learned in a conversation with friends that women do not menstruate when they are pregnant. She knew that her own cousin had already begun menstruating, and yet she had not; therefore, she was convinced that she herself was pregnant.

The girl's mother was upset by this. She also was taken aback by her ten year old daughter's concern with sexuality even before she had entered puberty. This parent was even more upset over the influence her daughter's peers apparently had over her. Most of all, what the mother could not face was that she needed to explain to her daughter about the relationship between intercourse and pregnancy.

Here lies the problem shared by parents since time immemorial. We remember that when we were growing up, few people ever talked to us about sex. Not your mother or father, your pastor, your teacher in school, or your neighbors next door—not anyone you had respect for. We know that many Catholic parents think that sex is frequently sinful and

1

feel ashamed talking about it. To make matters worse, we live in a society of instant communication which today includes frank and open discussion of sex and sexual issues. After the silence and negative attitudes of the past, we are being told to be open, positive and relaxed. The ten year old girl needs a mother who knows some facts about intercourse and can discuss them with her daughter without feeling frustrated and disgusted by this responsibility.

We know that over eighty percent of parents in our society want to talk to their own children about sex. They want to discuss more than the facts of reproduction. Most important is their ability to guide their children with attitudes and values which will help them grow into healthy, Christian young adults. In the papal encyclical *Familiaris Consortio* John Paul II stresses that "education must bring the children to a knowledge of and respect for the moral norms as the necessary and highly valuable guarantee for responsible personal growth in human sexuality." A basic principle of this teaching is that "the Church is firmly opposed to imparting sex information dissociated from moral principles." To help parents begin talking about sex with their children, we need first to clarify the difference between sex and sexuality.

When people hear the word "sex" they think of intercourse and reproduction. Often the word "sex" is used in two ways: (1) it labels genders, that is, whether a person belongs to the male or female gender; (2) it also refers to the physical part of the relationship. For example, "I had sex last night" usually refers to a physical, erotic, or genital relationship. But sexuality means something much broader. Sexuality includes all our experiences, our learnings, our knowledge, our dreams, our fantasies, our sexual experiences, and our relationships—the parts of our lives that have to do with being male or female. Sexuality begins from conception and continues into eternity. This understanding of sexuality is affirmed by the Vatican Congregation for Catholic Education which teaches: "Sexuality characterizes man and woman not only on the physical level, but also on the psychological and spiritual levels, making its mark on each of their expressions." This teaching makes the point that people who are "inclined to reduce sexuality to genital experience alone . . . devalue sex, as though by its nature men and women were defiled by it." The guidelines "intend to oppose such devaluation." The document states very clearly that the fundamental objective of sex education is to provide "adequate knowledge of the nature and importance of sexuality and the harmonious and integral development of the person toward psychological maturity, with full spiritual maturity in view, to which all believers are called."

We need to appreciate that sexual relationships need not, and most often do not, involve sex in its physical, genital aspect. Husbands and wives, parents and children, men and women, priests and religious—all these people are having sexual relationships in the sense that they are, in part, relating to each other as the male or the female each of them is. While genital sexual activity is an important aspect of some of our human relationships, it takes up a very small part of our waking time with a very small proportion of the people to whom we relate. Yet many parents worry about their children having genital sexual activity. Here is another struggle we cannot deny.

As parents and teachers in the Christian community, we believe that it is not desirable for teenagers to have intercourse. It's not only that there are 1.3 million pregnancies each year among teens, and several thousand new cases of venereal disease; it's also that, even if they were married, we know that teenagers are too young, too vulnerable, too available for exploitation. A shocking fact to many parents is that half of all young people in the United States will have intercourse in their teen years whether we like it or not. The reasons vary from one boy and girl to the next. In one school situation, a teacher remarked, "You know that girl in the eighth grade? I wouldn't be surprised if she gets pregnant before she graduates." When the teacher was asked if anyone was going to talk to the girl, the answer was, "We can't accuse her of anything; that would be rash judging. Anyway, there's a unit on dating coming up in three weeks for her class." In three weeks, she might already be pregnant!

Why do we wait for a crisis before we act? We know why teenage girls get pregnant. It's because they have sexual intercourse. What this young girl needs is someone to sit down and say to her, "I think you should know that I am concerned about you." We're not helping our young people whenever we moralize, or set rules, or just explain to them the facts of reproduction. We need to give them some messages, in advance, of pregnancy, such as the fact that it's all right to tell the boyfriend: "No!" If he's really a friend, he won't pressure you. We need to state the fact that almost ninety percent of teenage boys who make girls pregnant eventually abandon them. This includes those who marry to cover the pregnancy. Fifty percent of the boys abandon the girls immediately upon learning the girl is pregnant by saying, "How do I know it was me?" Most of the time, she knows, and, if he is honest, so does the boy.

The frightening reality is that only ten percent of the parents say anything about sex to their children. Too often, when children do ask questions, parents display such difficulty in expressing their feelings or attitudes that no one attempts to bring up the subject again. Parents often betray themselves. While they want to help their own children to progress rather than regress in sexual knowledge, attitudes and values, in reality too many allow their own sexual ignorance, anxieties, fears and shame to be passed on to their children. The Church's recent teaching on sex education is quite aware that "parents are often not sufficiently prepared to impart adequate sex education," and that sometimes "parents do not feel able to perform this duty." However, the Holy Father calls upon all parents to offer their children this education because he sees "the family as the best environment to accomplish the obligation of securing an education in sexual life." He understands how our culture has impoverished our vision of sexuality with selfishness, and he challenges parents to get involved in "a true formation not limited to the informing of the intellect, but paying attention to the will, to feelings and emotions." In his statement on the Christian family, John Paul asked parents to "aim firmly at a training in the area of sex that is truly and fully personal: for sexuality is an enrichment of the whole person—body, emotions and soul." This encouragement and confidence that the Church can offer parents in taking up their responsibility comes at a time of crisis in this generation.

The key element parents need to nurture in their children is the central message of the Gospel, in which St. John calls us "to love one another." This means caring for, as well as about, each other; we are called to be people of patience and understanding, and to be confidence builders. This can get pretty difficult in the everyday hectic life of a parent. Often we interpret the message of love in family life in terms of sending the kids to the dentist, keeping the refrigerator stocked with food, or driving them to another school function. Then again, it is hard being a manager, referee, judge and counselor all day long. So tensions build. These struggles are real, not imagined, but it is avoidance that leads to the most harm. In any case, such "household chaos" is pretty normal for all parents, and not limited to sensitive sexual topics. Our insensitivity, our indifference to taking on the responsibility of guiding our children in their sexual relationships is as great an evil as is our fear of promiscuity among them. Some groups warn that society's and the Church's preoccupation with sexual issues is a crisis that needs to be silenced and oppressed. However, the Vatican document explicitly states that "silence is not a valid way of conduct" because there are too many "hidden persuaders whose influence today is undeniable." Therefore, it is up to parents "to repair the harm caused by inappropriate and injurious interventions, but, above all, to opportunely inform their own children with a positive education." The risks involved in living the Christian life demand that parents look at the task of educating their children in sexuality and see it as an opportunity for grace. The guidelines "reaffirm that this aspect of education is first a work of faith for the Christian and a way to grace. Each aspect of sex education is inspired by faith and draws strength from it and from grace." The power of the Spirit is a gift from God given to enable the "faith-filled" to have the strength and courage to put aside past fears about their sexuality. The Spirit enables parents to grow in peace, joy, patience, goodness and fidelity. The power of the Spirit won't make parents perfect, but it can enable them to grow in the gifts of God. Here lies another real struggle for many people. How can we teach our young people about appropriate sexual relationships when we ourselves may have experienced failure and shame in our own sexual behavior?

Critics often blame their feelings of guilt on the teachings of the Church. However, the teaching Church is not static. The sending of the Spirit was intended to continue our spiritual development. Our spiritual development must be seen as an integral component of each person's spirituality. Spirituality is a yearning for union with God, which includes our sexuality as male or female, and therefore is a key element in our human personality. The lessons of Jesus Christ teach us to keep ourselves forever open to new knowledge, new understanding, and new opportunities. We are commanded to make the message of God's love for us a living reality, a part of our everyday experience. We know that society is starving for affection, for intimacy, for a message that speaks to the hearts of all men and women, hurt and angered as they may be by the guilt, the fear, the conflicts carried inside their hearts for so long. Jesus knew how to bring life back into the hearts of fearful and oppressed people. It was with words of hope, comfort, love, and encouragement that Jesus showed us how to mend broken lives with a message of forgiveness. He challenged his followers to do the same for each other. In regard to our sexual relationships, this is the love we want to pass on to our children. This is the love that as parents we want to express in gesture, word and touch in our homes for each other and for our children.

Only recently during this generation, there have been several official Church documents stressing the need "to carry out a positive work of sex education" to help children and adolescents. This ministry was strongly emphasized by the Council fathers in the *Declaration on Christian Education* (*Gravissimum Educationis*, 1966) which declared that "children and young people should be assisted in the harmonious development of their physical, moral and intellectual endowments. As they advance in years, they should be given positive and prudent sexual education."

In January 1974 the *Declaration on Certain Questions Concerning Sexual Ethics* was published by the Vatican Congregation for the Doctrine of the Faith which reaffirmed the Church's traditional teachings on morality and the role of parents as sex educators by stating: "They (parents) will prudently give them (children) information suited to their age; and they will assiduously form their wills in accordance with Christian morals."

In the *Apostolic Exhortation on the Family* (*Familiaris Consortio*, 1981) the Pope stated at one point: "In the context of a culture which seriously distorts or entirely misinterprets the true meaning of human sexuality because it separates it from its essential reference to the person, the Church more urgently feels how irreplaceable is its mission of presenting sexuality as a value and task of the whole person, created male and female in the image of God."

An increasing number of pastoral statements in the United States on national and diocesan levels have encouraged local parishes to initiate this new family ministry in human sexuality. The U.S. Catholic Conference published guidelines in 1981 which reaffirmed the Pope's teaching: "Parents have the right and the responsibility to provide guidance to their children about their sexual life within the attitudes that are appropriate in our Christian teaching. This ministry is a task for the Church at all times, which should be taking place in the home, the school, and in our parish communities."

Another 1981 statement issued by the bishops of New Jersey declared education in human sexuality to be "an important priority of Christian education in our respective dioceses."

Finally, the Congregation for Catholic Education in December 1983 reaffirmed the Holy Father's appeal to parents that "there is an urgent need to give positive and gradual affective sex education to children, adolescents and young adults." It calls upon "episcopal conferences to promote action in such an important ministry for the future of young people and the good of society." The Church's continued commitment to this ministry comes from the realization that we can no longer cover our children's eyes and ears to prevent them from getting information about sex. Too often ignorance and false modesty leads parents to tell untruths about sexual life, or to postpone telling truths until puberty, by which time children have heard society's false messages and will no longer hear what their parents are saying. Parents received this responsibility to share their faith in baptism. We know that young people do not grow up in a vacuum when it comes to learning values. The teachings of Christ serve as guidelines in our relationships with other people. Therefore, when it comes to sexual relationships, we believe it is a mistake not to tell young people what we stand for. We need to teach by our example. The Vatican document reaffirms this principle: "Christian parents must know that their example represents the most valid contribution in the education of their children." We need to show our young people how to express love, fidelity, responsibility, and chastity and how to accept differences and affirm other people in all our relationships. To be faith-filled means that we must respond honestly to all the questions our children have about their sexual natures. The Church's teaching since Vatican II regarding sex education has "affirmed the right of young people to receive an education adequate to their personal requirements."

Why should the Church become involved in this ministry? Because basically parents are seeking guidance and affirmation. They need to understand that it is devastating for an unprepared girl to experience her first menstruation when she thinks she is bleeding to death. That has been a horrible experience for too many women because no one prepared them for this normal event. People joke when they hear their seven year old describe how their baby brother or sister grew in mommy's tummy and came out like a bowel movement. "How cute," people say. However, where our children receive most of their sex education is not so cute or funny. It comes from television, records, magazines, advertisements, and their peers, and not from sources to be respected and trusted like trained teachers, the Church community and ourselves. Most of the messages about sex urge young people to buy, look and feel sexy. We must teach rather that all sex education needs to begin long before the young person's desire for designer jeans, even before the first step inside school. Sex education starts the moment a mother and father hold their newborn. It continues every time mom powders baby's bottom or dad changes a diaper. It's our reaction to their crying, their bowel movements, their burping and spitting and need for cuddling. Your child's sex education began with your delight or disappointment at the news whether it was a boy or a girl. What kind of messages do you think you have given your child? More important, what messages do you intend to provide as your newborn grows as a sexual person?

Many parents are apt to think of sex education only in terms of information about reproduction. But far more important are the attitudes that parents unconsciously express about sex, about themselves, or about each other as male or female. We know that children are constantly learning by observation, by being taught, or by experiencing what their culture and Church tradition consider desirable for males and females to be or to do. This concept of growth and development as a male or female is called the process of sexualization. In early sex education, parents' self-images, their role behaviors, and attitudes, their fear of or comfort with the erotic aspects of sex in their own lives—all these become important factors in the sexualization process of their children. It is during this process that children can develop happy, comfortable attitudes about themselves as male or female or negative and guilt-ridden feelings. Herein also lies another struggle. Too often parents wait for a crisis of adolescence to tackle the misinformation, fear, shame and confusion. Rather, young parents of the newborn need to accept and prepare themselves for the responsibility of providing sex education. Adolescence is too late to begin.

The Church has a distinct advantage over many secular institutions in that parents have confidence and trust in its moral guidance. Parents need the Christian community more than ever to support, respect, and teach them their unique roles as responsible sex educators. We must challenge any atmosphere of indifference. We have to recognize as a myth that any knowledge is harmful, that sexual information encourages sexual activity, and that today's sophisticated adolescents are already well informed. Research shows that none of this is true. We must commit ourselves to the truth. Before we can educate our children, we must seek and accept education for ourselves. The Vatican strongly supports "a solid cate-chetical preparation for adults on human love" as the foundation for the sex education of children. This does not presuppose that you are going to enjoy doing this or that you will feel comfortable learning, at least at first. Parenting means taking responsibility for many things that are not neat and easy, taking care of sick kids with diarrhea, changing smelly diapers, or learning how to control obscene language in the home. Becoming involved means that you have the choice of teaching your children well or poorly, so you might as well do the best possible job. Parents are their children's primary teachers about love for God and neighbor, and about sex, whether or not they know or accept this responsibility. Parents can never be the exclusive educators of their children, but they can be the most influential.

Here are some helpful guidelines for you as you read this book. First, be open to the possibility that there is information new to you that can enhance your life and help you be-come more enthusiastic, more compassionate, more ready and willing to respond to your children's questions about sex.

Second, this new learning requires effort on your part, and it is difficult to trust new people, new information and new methods. Anything really worthwhile in life is risky, but unless we put behind us our past fears, we may miss many opportunities to grow as Jesus intended us to become.

Third, some people press too hard. Their expectations are too high, and they expect themselves to be more knowledgeable, comfortable and spontaneous overnight. That's sim-ply not possible. We are not computers with unlimited capacities to record, process, and print our data. A computer cannot love. We can and must. Learning requires patience and understanding, as well as time for reflection and prayer. We need to accept ourselves, our attitudes and values, where we are now, excited that we are making a commitment to learn how to answer our children's questions honestly, clearly and with God's help.

Fourth, this book is not a version of the "big talk" about sex which you dreaded giving and were so glad when it was over. Instead, it is about the many small talks that should go on from day to day. Learning is part of a process that takes place gradually over many years. The process of sexualization includes many experiences that children have, beginning with their birth. Like any new work, parents, as they go along, will be rethinking, changing, ma-turing, and examining new ideas because God endowed us with wonderful, open minds.

Fifth, the book is designed to be used by individuals, couples, or parish or community discussion groups. We hope that whatever your situation, you will find someone to discuss and share new ideas with. If you are in a discussion group, we hope you will be made to feel comfortable enough to really participate, ask questions, and share your own experiences in the home. If you feel uneasy for a while, that's all right. Don't "fake it" if you would rather not participate in any of the discussion. Do only what you are comfortable with, but keep on growing.

Sixth, if your group is going to feel comfortable and really learn, you will need to have trust in each other's confidentiality. Some of you will, no doubt, wish to share some of your own personal experiences. In order to do this well, we need to accept and respect the feelings and experiences of others without judgment or criticism.

Seventh, along with confidentiality, lots of acceptance is needed. Each of us is a unique individual, and the opinions of each are going to be different from those of all others. In some instances, this will only be a nuance or shade of emphasis. In others, we may find differences that seem at first impossible to tolerate. But remember that we have come together to learn and to grow, and we hope that part of that growth will include accepting differences as well as similarities, and resisting the temptation to ridicule others. Finally, we know that life is meant to be serious, but not grim. So why not try to enjoy your study group and rediscover your playful side, which can help ease some of the tension when talking about sex.

Questions for Discussion

1. What thought in this section impressed you the most?
2. What in this section do you find most difficult to accept?
3. How would you define sexuality?
4. What is the role of our Church in sexuality education?
5. Which makes it more difficult to feel relaxed and open about sex—past negative attitudes or past lack of information?
6. Do you think our country reflects a Christian attitude toward sexual relationships? Why? Why not? What is a Christian attitude about sex?
7. What is your impression of the way fathers and/or mothers encourage their children to ask questions about sex?
8. What are some of the things you want your children to learn about sexuality?
9. How would you help to build the confidence of other parents in dealing with their children's sexuality?
10. What programs are available in your community which have the potential to build the sexual self-confidence of parents?

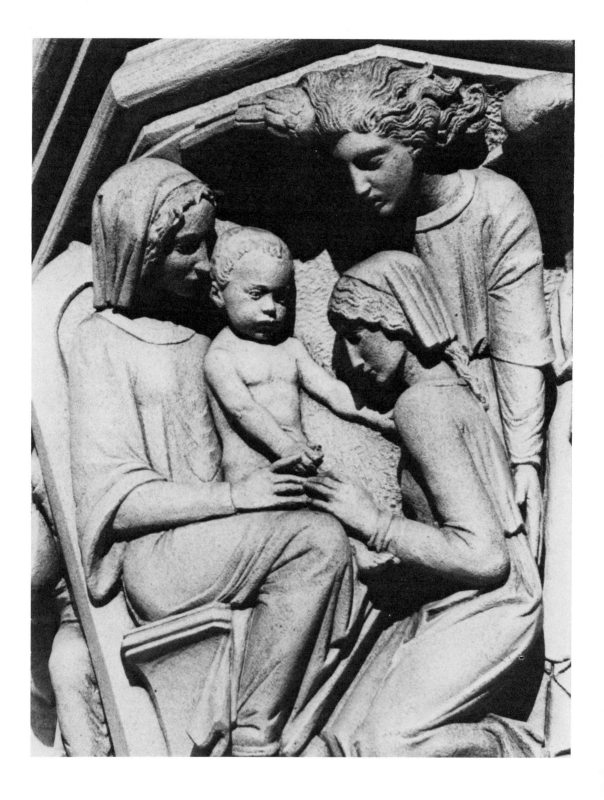

Church Tradition in Sexuality

Scientific advances in artificial contraception have created a crisis in sexual morality. The most recent discovery is a vaccine that will keep a woman infertile for three months. These advances strike at the basic guiding principle of the Catholic Church and religious sexual morality. All sexuality was considered to be ordained by God for the procreation of children. From the very beginning of life, all sexual activity was required to have childbearing as its primary end. Sexuality did serve other purposes such as strengthening the marriage bond or providing an outlet for biological drives. But these were considered not as important as reproduction. They were not at all valid without the intention of having children.

Being able to separate the reproductive goal of sexuality from the subordinate goals causes changes. People might now understand and live their sexuality in new ways. Sexual activity may have new meanings. It could now have a different purpose for a different good. But should it? Is such a change in tune with God's will? Could or should the Church change some very fundamental teachings?

Many people think that the crisis in sexual morality involves only birth control. But there is much more. Two questions form the foundation of this problem. What is the real purpose of human sexuality? And how do we discover this purpose? People's search for these answers leads to other questions. Is sex really good in itself? Or is it just given to sinful mankind because God is aware of our weakness? How should we think about ourselves and others as sexual persons? How should we judge various sexual activities? How do we know what is right and wrong sexually? Should the Church have the authority to tell us what to do? Or should each person depend upon his or her own conscience? If each person must decide, then what basic rules can help in these decisions? How can people stay honest and unbiased in making decisions about sexuality?

Our society has, for the most part, abandoned the original and truly Christian view of sexuality. Studies in various human sexuality reports make it clear that most people in the United States do not follow the traditional Christian teaching in their sexual lives. But that is no reason for Christians to change their own understanding of sexuality. Morality is not built on public opinion polls or majority vote.

We can still look within the Christian tradition for answers to the fundamental questions. But we must look more closely than before. We must look past the human weakness of interpretation. We must look beyond what was "common" opinion in past ages. We must look again to see the truths that have been there, but missed, all along. Our search can be divided into four basic parts: a more careful and informed reading of Scripture, a more honest look at the historical tradition, an analysis of modern research into human life, and a Christian concept of sexuality as outlined in the most recent Vatican document on sex education.

I. A New Reading of Scripture

The New Testament, particularly the Gospels, says little about sexual morality. The Old Testament does give specific rules for some sexual activities. But for some sexual issues, there is no scriptural text or story that can give us clear guidance. These issues are: masturbation, pornography, obscene jokes and language, nude bathing, nudist colonies, premarital sex, artificial contraception, male or female sterilization, artificial insemination, test tube babies, and surrogate motherhood. It is possible to find clear condemnation of freely chosen homosexual relations in both the Old and New Testaments (Lev 20:13; Rom 1:27). But these are thought to be linked to pagan religious practices and show no awareness of the condition of homosexual orientation that from earliest childhood is irreversible. Both Testaments have condemnations of adultery (Lev 20:10; Mk 10:19), but the reasons for the condemnations vary. The Gospels speak of Jesus' rejection of divorce and remarriage, but St. Matthew allows for an exception (Mk 10:1–12; Lk 18:10; Mt 19:9).

St. Paul is the most outspoken New Testament author on sexual morality. He clearly rejects prostitution, orgies, adultery, and voluntary homosexuality. He also favors celibacy over marriage. But he allows divorce and remarriage in one special case (1 Cor 7:15–16). Nowhere does the New Testament even suggest that procreation is the purpose of sexuality and marriage.

We find that no issue of sexual morality can be settled simply by quoting a text. But that does not mean that the revelation of God's word in Scripture leaves us without any help for working out a sexual morality. Scripture does help us with three basic understandings about sexuality: a proper attitude toward sexuality; the purpose of sexuality; the importance of interior intentions in all sexual behavior.

A. ATTITUDES TOWARD SEXUALITY

One clear and consistent teaching of the Scriptures is that God created us male and female. He created sexual beings and sexuality. And, when he looked at what he had made, he said it was very good. God meant what he said. We are the very best of creation—not only as infants with rosy cheeks, or as children with cute smiles, but also as teenagers, grown-ups and old people. In the second creation story, the only thing not good is for the human person to be alone. God quickly remedied this with the creation of man and woman. Human beings are meant from this very creation to be male and female. Sexuality is a part of God's good creation. It is as man and woman together that humanity is "in the image and likeness of God." Sexuality is not dirty, nor an embarrassment or a mistake. Rather, it is a gift and a blessing.

It is not only the creation stories in the Book of Genesis that display this positive attitude toward sexuality. The Old Testament is full of sexual imagery used to describe the relationship between God and his chosen people. The Song of Songs is an explicit hymn in praise of sexual attraction and love. This same attitude is confirmed in the Synoptic Gospels. Nowhere is it contradicted in the New Testament except for a few passages in Paul. We'll explain these shortly.

A careful, critical reading of Scripture has made it clear that the puritanical, Jansenistic and Victorian attitudes toward sexuality were mistaken ones, even though they were common in the history of Christian faith. Writers of both the Old and New Testaments were well aware that sexuality, like all dimensions of human life, can be broken by sin and often misused, as can any and all others of God's good gifts (Sam 12:1–15; 1 Cor 5:1–8). It still remains a great gift and blessing of God in which we can rejoice.

It is easy for us to affirm and defend in words such a positive attitude, but history testifies that it is not easy to practice this in our daily lives. Various puritanical tendencies have infected Christian thinking from the earliest days of the Church. Christian hostility toward the body, toward women, and toward all things sexual has often been exaggerated. But there is no question that negative attitudes have crept into Christian thought from a variety of external sources that are completely contradictory to Scripture. It is important to find out why this has been the case.

Two basic factors have opened the door for all the other influences to take hold. One is St. Paul's clear preference for celibacy over marriage. This ideal has been institutionalized in the Church in the form of celibacy and virginity required of clergy and religious. The religious life has come to be thought of as a better or more excellent state than marriage. Intentionally or not, this preference for celibacy has tended to treat marriage as a second class form of Christian life. This notion is confirmed in St. Paul's statement: "It is better to marry than to burn." Almost from the outset, Christian sexual morality took on a negative cast. As a result, no adequate Christian theology of sexuality and marriage has ever been developed.

The second door-opener to the myriad of negative attitudes is probably the most basic, and probably strongly influenced by St. Paul. Throughout history, mankind has often experienced the disruptive nature of sexual attraction and sexual love. Sexual desire can and does cause both personal and social problems. It is a source of both joy and sorrow, pleasure and pain, life and death, community and chaos. It seems to draw some people away from God as readily as it draws others close to him. This ambiguity has been the experience of many Christians. They have put their stamp on the Christian tradition by the influence of their writings. St. Augustine of the fourth century is the most notable of such figures. Uncomfortable experiences with sex often caused people to be wary, and to adopt a negative and ambiguous attitude toward all aspects of sexuality. These people's central concern was not to experience the goodness of God's gift to the fullest. They spent great amounts of energy trying to control its expression. As with all ambiguous realities, there is a tendency to move toward extremes. People have tended to adopt attitudes either of extreme hostility toward sexuality or of complete abandon and indiscriminate acceptance of it.

It is here that a new or renewed reading of Scripture is essential. Paul's preference for celibacy and other supportive statements (Mt 19:12) can be better understood with a little research. It is found that it is not simply celibacy or virginity that is the ideal. Rather, Paul urges celibacy embraced for the sake of the Kingdom of God. Both Paul and the Synoptic Gospels are clear that such a calling is not for everyone and so is not an ideal for everyone. We must also remember that the early Church was awaiting Christ's return and expected it at any moment. In this circumstance, the energy spent on managing sexual relationships, and procreation as well, might better be spent on preparing for the second coming of Jesus. Contemporary authors are careful to make clear that marriage and consecrated celibacy need one another and enhance the value of each other. Where marriage is demeaned as a way of life, so also is the value of celibate commitment and sacrifice. When the celibate commitment is demeaned, then so also is the great human good of sexual love.

There is a second consideration that arises from Paul's preference for celibacy for the sake of the Kingdom. It is that there is something more important and more fundamental in human life than sexual fulfillment and the blessings of children and family. Paul is very clear that all things must become secondary to the Kingdom of God. Sexuality has frequently been made into an idol itself, worshiped with religious fervor. Sexual cults were part of many early religions, including those surrounding the Israelites of the Old Testament. The writers of the Old Testament were familiar with these pagan cults and fought their influence constantly. Sexual activity, as part of pagan religious worship, was still present in the time of Paul, and he attempted to protect the early Christian communities from them. Even today we can accept that, for some, sex has become an idol, given worship beyond all else. Paul places sexuality in the service of the Kingdom. Others have misread him and gone to the extreme of denying any value of sex.

In practice, a careful reading of Scripture provides an attitude toward sexuality that reminds us of its great good as well as its power. This attitude also shows us that sexuality is by no means the highest or ultimate good. The meaning of life is not to be found in sexuality.

Sex is neither demonic nor divine. It is neither to be feared nor worshiped, but turned to the service of God's Kingdom.

B. THE PURPOSE OF SEXUALITY

A second insight about sexual morality we can gain from Scripture concerns the purpose of sexuality in human life. From the time of St. Augustine (fourth century) until the Second Vatican Council, the Church has taught that the primary purpose of sexuality is the procreation of children. In this way it served a social good, the continuation of the human species. Other possible good effects of sexuality were acknowledged. But these were all secondary and subordinate to the good of procreation. This teaching is not supported by Scripture. Neither the Gospels, which refer back to Genesis, nor the writings of Paul explain the meaning of sexuality as primarily for procreation. They do not deny the procreative function, but neither do they define it as the sole purpose of sexuality. The importance of our sexual natures is seen in forming the community of male and female. A new reality is found when a man leaves his father and mother and clings to his wife. In the second creation account of Genesis, before male and female are created, God finds one thing not good. It is not good for a person to be alone. Only as man and woman, Adam and Eve, are the persons able to fill up each other's loneliness. Of all creation, only the human person is able to be partner and helpmate to the other. In the Synoptic Gospels, when Jesus explains why God created male and female, the reason is clearly that two should become one (Mk 10:5–10). Of course, this union is given the command and the blessing to be fruitful and multiply. This union is to serve life; it does have procreative meaning. But that purpose is not mentioned as being the only or even the most important reason for humanity's creation as male and female.

St. Paul sees the union of male and female as a means of mutual sanctification and a sign of the union of Christ with his Church (1 Cor 7:14–16; Eph 5:21–23). This is now called the "unitive function" of sexuality as a force that draws people together. Now we can look back and see that it is this unitive function, not procreation, that has always been stressed in Scripture. It is the union, the two becoming one, that the Bible points to as the central purpose of sexuality. It would seem, then, that that purpose must become the yardstick for what is morally acceptable in sexual behavior.

This does not deny or overlook the high value given to procreation in Scripture. Children are clearly thought of as a blessing. They are the expected fruit of the sexual union, a gift from God. Female barrenness or deformation or mutilation of the male sex organs is looked upon as a curse and a humiliation. Elizabeth, the mother of John the Baptist, is a familiar example of a woman's joy at pregnancy achieved where none was thought possible (Lk 1:25). There are numerous, similar stories throughout the Old Testament. But childbearing and rearing is not an obligation of nature in the Scriptures. Rather, it is an obligation of the covenant. In the New Testament, the new covenant, it is an obligation that may be overridden for the sake of the Kingdom.

C. THE IMPORTANCE OF INTERIOR INTENTIONS

The third insight into sexual morality that we find in Scripture is the strong emphasis Jesus placed upon the intentions of the heart for a genuine morality (Mt 5:20–30; Mk 7:14–23). The need for us to understand the emphasis on interior intentions has been shown recently by the worldwide reaction to a statement made by Pope John Paul II. He commented that "if a man gazes on his wife lustfully, he has already committed adultery with her in his heart." Marriage is not an excuse for wrong intentions.

Jesus emphasizes in his teaching that the most crucial element in morality is not the external act, but the inner intention from which the act comes. On what is a person's heart set? It is not what comes from the outside that corrupts us, but rather what comes from within. Calling one's brother a fool and lusting after even a wife in one's heart are declared to be as morally corrupting as the external acts of murder and adultery.

The importance of intentions can also be shown in positive ways. Jesus' basic moral demand was a call for conversion (Mk 1:15). "What must we do to be saved?" "Repent and believe in the good news." The primary demand is not for a change of behavior so much as for a change of mind and heart; then the behavior will automatically follow. Jesus asks us to turn away from the intention to serve ourselves. He asks us to be intent upon seeking first the Kingdom of God and the service of neighbor. In the Scriptures, in John's Gospel and First Epistle, and in the writings of Paul, love of God and of neighbor exhaust and fulfill the whole law (Jn 13:34–35; 1 Jn 2:10; 1 Cor 13:1–13). The essence of morality is found in what the heart loves, in what the human person interiorly intends. While love is not the only motive Jesus gives for moral action, it is certainly the highest. All are invited to strive for this. This does not mean that morality is complete by having good intentions or simply meaning well; it does show that the morality Jesus outlined for us cannot be wholly found within the limits of the written law. No list or description of sexual acts, no matter how long or complete, can encompass the sexual morality or non-morality of the Christian life. In practice, this means that Gospel morality demands full personal responsibility. Each individual is responsible for choices and decisions made and carried out in full conscience.

II. Historical Tradition

From the beginning, the Church has put great emphasis on "what is believed everywhere, at all times, by all." This formed a foundation for judging doctrine. The possibility of changing a teaching that was thought to have such tradition behind it was almost unthinkable. But a study of history often shows that such traditions were usually less uniform, less consistent, and less certain than was once thought. Studies by scholars such as John Noonan's on contraception, John Connery's on abortion, and John Boswell's on homosexuality show the wide variation of acceptance in the tradition on sexual teaching. These studies also show that some teachings were based on incomplete or untrue biological, psychological, or philosophical knowledge. More correct knowledge in these cases is available to us today. A complete explanation of the tradition of sexual morality is too large for this essay. Three examples can give a clear picture of the problems tradition has had in sexual morality. They are the role of women, the behavior of animals, and the knowledge of biology.

A. THE ROLE OF WOMEN

Almost all historical writings on sexual morality were written by males, for males, about males. The recognition of such prejudice in most traditions does not mean that their teachings must be wrong. This should not be used as an easy excuse for finding fault with our ancestors in the faith. But it does, at least, call those traditions into serious question that see woman as the property of man, and an object of his lust. An understanding of woman as the created helpmate of man, equal in the image of God, finds problems with some traditions. The virtue of chastity, as the right understanding and use of sexuality, is the equal responsibility of both men and women. The meaning of chastity cannot be different for men and for women. The "double standard" can find no protection in Genesis. Still, what it means to honor the full human status of woman is only slowly beginning to be understood. The growth in understanding and respect for women has had a large impact on sexual morality. One area of this is now seen in law. It is possible, and now illegal in some states, for a husband to rape his wife. Marriage may include a type of right to the body of the spouse, but not with the use of force or violence. It is possible, and morally wrong, as Pope John Paul II reminded us, for a husband to lust after his wife in his heart.

This new growth in the understanding of the role of women also challenges the sexual morality of females. Female sexuality is not to be used as a weapon of seduction or manipulation. Neither should it be used by men or women as a reward and punishment mechanism. When sex is used as a power play between men and women, it loses its meaning and power in life. The new understanding of women demands new responsibility by both men and women to contradict the subtle forms of sexual manipulation. The sexual relationship leading to the union of two in one flesh can only sustain its moral integrity if it is an equal and mutually caring relationship. It is time to stop talking about the obligation of a wife to submit to her husband's advances. Such an obligation, as Paul told the Corinthians (1 Cor 7:4–5), can only be a mutual one.

B. THE BEHAVIOR OF ANIMALS

One of the most persistent habits in the tradition of Western morality has been to equate what is immoral with what is unnatural. This is relatively harmless if we are clear about what we mean by natural and unnatural. We must also be quite clear about how we decide the difference. But historical studies show us that this has not been the case in Western tradition. Modern students of animal behavior are not the first to think they can learn something about human nature by observing what animals do. Thomas Aquinas was one of the most influential shapers of the Catholic moral tradition. He was quite sure that anyone could discover what was natural—and therefore morally correct—sexual behavior simply by observing what animals do. Many of his conclusions about sexual morality were based upon this belief and upon what, apparently, he thought he observed. Thomas was convinced that animals did not masturbate, did not engage in homosexual activity, and did not seek out species other than their own to satisfy their sexual instincts. Hence, he concluded that masturbation, homosexuality, and bestiality were unnatural and, so, immoral. But animals do, in fact, do the things Aquinas said they did not do. His observations were faulty and inadequate—and thus, perhaps also, his conclusions. If homosexual activity is natural in the sense that some animals do engage in it, is it therefore morally right? More important, while human sexuality has points in common with animal sexuality, it is altogether a different moral matter precisely because it is a human activity. It is an activity of conscious, free, rational persons, which gives it a different meaning in every way.

It is true that we can learn many things by observing animals and the principles of nature's operation. However, we cannot learn what is humanly right or wrong from such observations. If we must then move away from Aquinas' understanding of the natural moral law, shouldn't we also move away from his conclusions about sexual morality? It would seem impossible not to. Aquinas ranked sexual sins from worst to least, according to whether they were more or less unnatural. In his ranking, masturbation was judged to be a more serious sin than adultery or even rape. The use of artificial contraception was a more serious sin than fornication. From any perspective of responsible behavior today, this ranking is certainly wrong. The crisis in sexual morality continues.

C. THE KNOWLEDGE OF BIOLOGY

For most of the history of humankind, knowledge of the human reproductive system was seriously incomplete. Until fairly recent times, people thought that the male "seed" contained the whole human being. The female womb was regarded as simply the field in which the seed was planted to grow to ripeness. The male was seen as having the "active" role in procreation, and the female a passive role. This idea was carried over into the traditional active and passive roles of males and females in sexual intercourse. Infertility was considered a completely female problem. It was often regarded as a curse and as more than adequate grounds for divorce, something that is still true in some places today.

Given this misunderstanding of the procreative process, it is easy to see why artificial contraception, masturbation, coitus interruptus, and abortion all had the same moral status, often being equated with murder. It is easy to see why the primary purpose of sexuality was thought to be procreation. It is also easy to see why sexual intercourse during pregnancy was considered senseless and wrong. The same would be true of intercourse after the female menopause. Who plants a seed in a field that has already been planted, or in a field known to be infertile?

Several scientific discoveries about the process of procreation have greatly increased our understanding of it, i.e., the existence and role of the female ovum, the physiology of the menstrual cycle, and the fact that a typical male ejaculation contains 400,000 to 2,000,000 spermatozoa, any one of which is capable of fertilizing an ovum and creating a new human being. In short, with knowledge of modern biology, it is not even possible to think as our ancestors once thought. Who today could give masturbation and abortion the same moral value, even while thinking they are both morally wrong? Once again, just knowing how and why the historical tradition believed as it did about sexual morality makes us question those conclusions and the teaching of tradition. This does not mean that we should abandon all traditional teaching. But it does cause a crisis in our understanding. Either a new base for the teaching must be found, or the teaching must be re-evaluated.

III. The Social Sciences

The social sciences have made great strides in our understanding of ourselves. Many people feel that these findings are not relevant to Christian faith. Others believe that this new body of knowledge only adds to the challenge that secular culture makes to our faith. There is very little need felt to take these findings into account in working out a sexual morality. The Kinsey Reports may be interesting and informative about what people actually did sexually, but they really had nothing to offer about what people *should* do sexually. Statistics are no basis for morality. To take another example, it might be helpful, from a practical point of view, to know that about six out of one hundred people have an exclusive homosexual orientation. But that knowledge will not decide the question about the morality of homosexual behavior. The fact that something is the case does not mean that it necessarily ought to be. Something more than statistics is needed. However, the findings of the empirical social sciences should be given close examination. There is undoubtedly some link between these and Christian sexual morality. The Christian faith makes a claim to truth. It believes that truth is ultimately one since the author of all truth is one. In this way it cannot afford to ignore truth from any source. All students of human behavior must be heard and evaluated. Truly, some new findings may cause new crises in sexual morality. Two particular issues will serve to illustrate this: masturbation and homosexuality.

MASTURBATION

The question of what to do about masturbation can become confusing to many parents. The Church's official teaching is that masturbation is wrong and should be avoided.

> Masturbation, according to Catholic doctrine, constitutes a grave moral disorder principally because it is the use of the sexual faculty in a way which essentially contradicts its finality, not being at the service of love and life according to the design of God (*Educational Guidance in Human Love*, 1983, par. 99).

On the other hand, modern psychology tells us that masturbation is a normal part of life, a way of relieving sexual and other tensions (*Human Sexuality*, James B. McCary, 1978, p. 150). It has been known for many years that there are no physical dangers inherent in masturbation.

These seemingly conflicting views can cause frustration and alienation for parents who are trying to do the right things for their children. To provide some insight we would like parents to consider several points. First, exactly what are the Church and modern psychology talking about when they use the word masturbation? There would seem to be a world of difference between conscious, purposeful, genital manipulation accompanied by well-formed sexual fantasies of older people and the simple exploration of one's body shape and physical sensation in infants. Between these seemingly opposite ends, psychology tells us that there is a whole range of meaning, purpose and control involved in genital touching.

Second, parents need to put a little effort into really understanding what is going on in their child's life when the question of masturbation arises. This needs to be matched with the question of moral responsibility or sin. Does the behavior have the three requirements for sin: serious matter, full understanding and control and conscious choice? This consideration of sin is not the only base on which parents should decide what to allow or not allow their children to do. But it can certainly help parents form their own personal attitudes toward their children's sexual behavior. Parents who for example angrily shout words of disgust at a child who is found touching his or her genitals are certainly concerned more with their own sexual attitudes and fear of sin than with the child's present moral condition and needs. As parents, we need to be more in control of the very strong positive or negative images we pass on to our children about their bodies both verbally and non-verbally. The best influences we can share with a child at a young age are images about our bodies conveyed with gentleness and mature understanding. A child at this early age of sexual development is intellectually unable to comprehend the moral implications until a later age. Parents who are uneasy when their child is touching his or her genitals can best teach the boundaries that are acceptable in their home with gentle and kind instructions. If we react very critically, are sharp in our remarks, express anger and disgust over their behavior, then we are teaching the child that his or her body is bad and evil, and, in essence, showing little respect and understanding for the primary Gospel message that what God created is good, and that includes our whole body. It is essential that in our teaching, we should not be violent in dealing with the sensual development of the child. Many studies indicate that interference in the child's sensual development is the primary cause for severe problems in relationships with other adults in later life (James Anthony *et al.*, 1984).

Along with understanding the meaning and purpose of genital exploration or self-pleasuring for the child at his or her own developmental stage, parents also need to be very clear on the attitudes and values about sexuality, bodies and sin they wish to convey. Children very easily absorb negative attitudes. Early feelings of guilt and shame about bodies and sexuality can cause less than healthy moral and emotional development for later life. How can the child cope with the conflicting messages of his own internal developmental program that says "Learn about your body," our spoken message that says, "God made your body beautiful and good," and our unspoken attitude that says, "When you touch yourself there, you're a bad kid"? Parents need to be consistent in the messages they give. And messages to young children should strongly emphasize the God-given goodness of our created bodies.

> A child's discovery of sexual parts of the body should be approached positively,
> and touching, which at this level is based primarily on curiosity and some sense

of pleasure, should not be condemned or considered unnatural. For the child, this is a beneficial and important learning process of discovering not only who God created, but also what God created (*Education in Human Sexuality for Christians*, USCC, 1981, p. 22).

As children mature and approach and enter puberty, sexual self-stimulation takes on new, morally responsible meanings. As children learn to understand the purpose and right use of human genital expression they should be taught that our sexuality should be placed "at the service of love and life according to the design of God" (*Educational Guidance in Human Love*, par. 99). As parents attempt to guide their children they should remember:

> . . . from an educational point of view, it is necessary to consider masturbation and other forms of eroticism as symptoms of problems much more profound, which provoke sexual tension that the individual seeks to resolve by recourse to such behavior. Pedagogic action therefore should be directed more to the causes than to the direct repression of the phenomenon (*Educational Guidance in Human Love*, 1983, par. 99).

The Church is charging parents to guide their children through adolescent masturbation not by condemnation and threats, but by active, positive teaching about the other-centered nature of our sexuality. Parents should strive with their adolescents to resolve the "growing pains" of peer pressure, media promises, the drive for independence, acceptance and love that turn the adolescent inward and foster habitual masturbation for relief of these stresses.

The Church, in stating that masturbation is a "grave moral disorder," is not forsaking or condemning the vast majority of people, who at some time in their lives masturbate (Kinsey *et al.*, 1948–1953). Rather, it is offering a challenge to be truly other-centered and loving with every facet of our sexual natures. The Church offers understanding that people are not always in complete control of their actions, especially adolescents.

As parents, we need to be gentle in dealing with our children on this issue. We should reflect the loving parental nature of God in guiding and teaching, rather than punishing and criticizing. By encouraging children in prayer, the sacraments, social action and true Christian growth we will develop in them the lifestyles of spiritual development and sexual self-esteem that make tension-relieving masturbation unnecessary.

Homosexuality

What can we say to homosexuals about their sexuality that will be spiritually helpful and in keeping with Christian faith and morality? Studies in the field of human sexuality have discovered a homosexual orientation that is apparently irreversible. There is a difference between a person who engages in homosexual activity and someone who is born with a genuine homosexual orientation. The cause of this orientation is still unknown and under intensive research. There is little doubt that homosexual acts are condemned in both the Old and New Testaments as unnatural and abominable in the sight of God. The persistent teaching of the Church reaffirmed by the Vatican document on sex education states that homosexual behavior cannot be "morally justified." It clearly lacks any procreative potential. But both the Scriptures and tradition speak of homosexuality as if it were a freely chosen way of behavior. The Church's continued advice and admonition is to change their behavior. It has already been cited that sexual practices, including homosexuality, were often a part of pagan religious worship in both the Old Testament and early New Testament times. This would greatly reinforce the repulsiveness of such acts in the eyes of the Jewish people and early Christians.

Now, studies in human sexuality have found that our sexual orientation is set long before the age of personal responsibility. In many if not most cases, this orientation is irreversible by any methods presently known to human beings. As a result, it seems clear that we are dealing with something very different from what St. Paul condemned.

The recent Vatican document addressed this issue by offering this teaching: "Pastorally, homosexuals must be received with understanding and supported in the hope of overcoming their personal difficulties and their social maladaption." However, "their culpability will be judged with prudence." The U.S. bishops issued a statement on homosexuality in their 1976 pastoral *To Live in Christ Jesus* by teaching: "Some persons find themselves through no fault of their own to have a homosexual orientation. Homosexuals, like everyone else, should not suffer from prejudice against their basic human rights. They have a right to respect, friendship and justice. Homosexual activity, however, as distinguished from homosexual orientation is morally wrong. . . . Because heterosexuals can usually look forward to marriage, and homosexuals, while their orientation continues, might not, the Christian community should provide them with a special degree of pastoral understanding and care."

IV. Christian Concept of Sexuality

The new Vatican statement on sex education stresses parental involvement as the most important contribution in the education of their children. Fundamental guidelines for sex education are presented in a document, released December 1, 1983 by the Vatican Congregation for Catholic Education, and entitled *Educational Guidance in Human Love*. The guidelines oppose devaluation of sexuality, but indicate that the reason may be found in society's tendency to reduce sexuality to genital experience alone. It is significant that the Vatican is supporting and encouraging sex education. For in past tradition, Pope Pius XI had condemned it, specifically the programs in his day which offered information of "a naturalist character, precociously and indiscriminately imparted." However, he did support a positive sex education "on the part of those who have received from God the educational mission." This positive value of sex education indicated by Pius XI was greatly enriched and encouraged by Vatican II. The document emphasizes that love is to be the characteristic of authentic sex. The purpose of appropriate sexual communion and the fundamental objective of this education has to be personal and spiritual maturity. "Sexuality, oriented, elevated, and integrated by love . . . is achieved in the full sense only with the realization of affective maturity."

Sexual intercourse has a twofold value, according to this teaching: an intimate communion of love between the couple and the fostering of children. In the several comments where these two values are presented, it is the unity that is placed ahead of fecundity. Augustine, Aquinas and Pius XI had ranked them in reverse order.

The new Vatican document states: "Love and fecundity are meanings and values of sexuality which include and summon each other in turn and cannot therefore be considered as either alternatives or as opposites." This harmony of the unitive and procreative values offers families a positive Christian perspective supporting the need for a balance between sexual intimacy and responsible parenting. The teaching is understanding of family life when it explains how arduous and demanding a fully human integration of genitality, eroticism and love really is. However, instead of blaming society for making this goal practically unattainable, it supposes that, although not many attain it fully, more people than we might imagine reach it reasonably well.

Sex education is essentially a responsibility of parents, to guide children in moral values: "Respect for life in the womb and, in general, respect for people of every age and condition have great importance." The role of the parent is to help the young "to understand, appreciate and respect these fundamental values of existence." While parents carry the primary responsibility as educators, "the school, parish and other ecclesial institutions are called to collaborate with the family." It is significant that the Vatican document states that "a solid catechetical program for adults on human love establishes the foundations for the sex education of children."

Another fundamental teaching affirmed by the document is preparation of the young for marriage which "aspires to sustain and strengthen the chastity proper to the engaged in preparation for conjugal life viewed in a Christian manner and to the specific mission which the married have among the people of God." Therefore, in order to live their sexuality and to carry out their responsibilities in accord with God's plan, young people should be made knowledgeable about natural methods of regulating fertility, and they should learn why artificial contraception does not harmonize "with responsible marriage, full of love and open to life."

This document seriously challenges sex education programs today which give "excessive weight to simple information, at the expense of the other dimensions of sex education." The many positive and supportive statements from the Vatican for sex education gives hope to the many families who have been struggling with this issue on their own. What is needed on the local parish level to carry out this responsibility is commitment and trust "of parents, of Christian communities and of educators" for action "for the future of young people and the good of society."

As we close this review of the history and tradition of the Church's teaching on sexual morality, we need to reflect on an important dimension of spiritual growth. Mystics describe it as the need to "flee," referring, for example, to Christ's journey to the mountains to pray.

However, this flight was not perceived as running away from the world, but as what we like to call the "flight to health." In order for us to grow as mature Christians in our sexual development, we will need to "flee," to disown those attitudes that oppose the goodness of our bodies, our sexual humanity. This "flight to health" requires a constant effort to integrate accurate information about our sexual lives with the healthy, compassionate attitude of God and the teaching of Scripture and Church tradition regarding human sexuality. This "flight to health" requires many of us to take the risk to rediscover and reaffirm the many positive messages found on sexuality in our Catholic tradition. Too little has been said about how people can live out their sexuality in a positive, joyful way.

Questions for Discussion

1. What factors have contributed to our modern crisis in sexual morality?
2. If morality is not built on majority vote or public opinion polls, then what *is* it built on?
3. "Our society has, for the most part, abandoned the truly Christian view of sexuality." Illustrate this statement by contrasting behaviors and attitudes of modern society with modern Christian behaviors and attitudes.
4. Why do you think some truths about sexuality have been missed by others in the past? Give examples of this.
5. In what ways does Scripture affirm the goodness of our sexuality?
6. How did negative attitudes toward sexuality creep into Christian thought? Name or describe some false beliefs and some misinterpretations.
7. What function of sexuality is stressed in Scripture? How is this related to other functions?
8. In what way does the importance of interior intentions, stressed in Scripture, demand personal responsibility? How does this relate to law as part of sexual morality?
9. How have some traditions, based on faulty or biased knowledge, affected our sexual morality today?
10. How does the study of Scripture, together with modern biological and social science, provide perspectives on such sexual questions as homosexuality and masturbation?
11. How does our concept of love either help or hinder our development of a sexual morality?
12. Where can you turn for personal help with questions about sexual morality?
13. How is the availability of correct information from reliable sources of primary importance to teens?
14. How can parents cope with older teens' maturational needs to take risks and try out new situations?

15. Where do teens ultimately get their values? How can parents remain influential in this area?
16. What are the most important needs of older teens? How can parents help to see that these needs are met?
17. Give examples of how important communication is between parents and children at each stage of development.

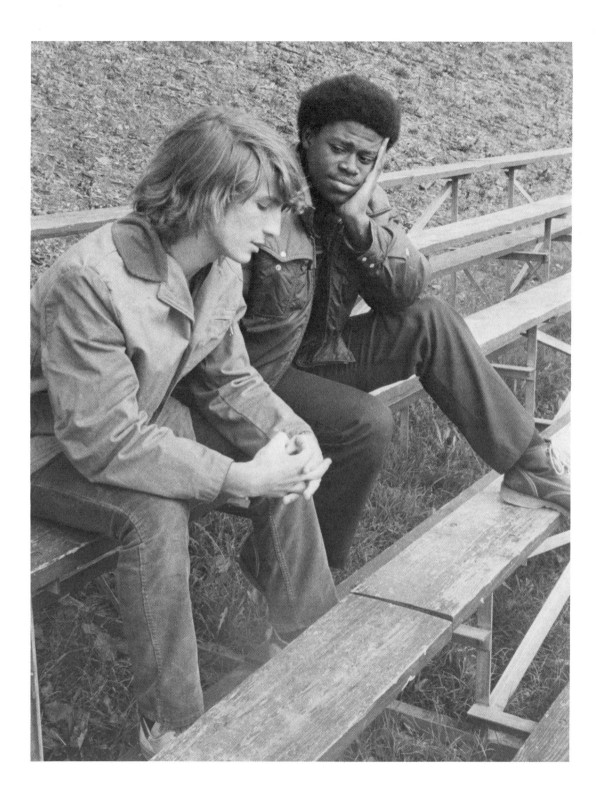

Sexual Myths

Some youngsters were given a homework assignment to ask everyone at home this question: "Where did you come from?" So one ambitious young girl went to her mom who replied, "The doctor brought me home in his little black bag." Not quite satisfied, she decided to ask her dad where he came from. He said: "Actually, the stork brought me home." Disturbed by this answer, she asked her grandma who she knew always told the truth. Grandma replied, "My dear child, everyone knows it's the angels who brought us here." So this little girl went back to school and gave this report: "I have discovered that there has not been a normal birth in my family for three generations."

Few parents are aware of how much a child's most lasting sex education takes place before he or she first steps into school. Actually, this education is based not so much on directly received information as on attitudes learned from parents, from other people, and, unfortunately, from television. These attitudes can be compassionate, understanding, and accepting as often as they can be prejudiced, dehumanizing, and shame-filled. Whether positive or negative, parents are constantly passing on sexual attitudes to their children, all the time, with or without words, in all kinds of ways.

We quickly discover that children always have questions about sex, whether we want them to or not. Despite that, what is important is that your child be able to depend on you always to tell the absolute truth. For, very crucially, this will protect the child from potential harm as well as from possible sexual dysfunction later in life, both of which have resulted, many times, from the untruths and myths passed around by children or perpetrated by adults.

27

We need not shy away from many opportunities that could provide openings for discussing sexuality or from raising questions about sex that our children may be longing to ask but are afraid to bring up. We are obliged, for their sakes, to teach the truth and put aside many of the old myths that are obstacles to enjoying the goodness of our embodied natures. We must perpetuate attitudes of respect for all life, tolerance of differences, acceptance of the pleasures our bodies hold, and willingness to share the truth. We want our children to be able to say to their friends with pride, "My dad and mom told me about the goodness of my body, and I can ask them anything!"

Parental Concerns

MYTH 1: *Teaching young children about their sexuality is harmful to their emotional growth.*

Knowledge is not harmful. Rather, our attitudes, values, and beliefs form the framework which influences a child's emotional impressions and reactions. Make no mistake—sexual information and misinformation are taking place all the time. Children are learning from a variety of sources what may or may not agree with our own sexual attitudes and beliefs or even be correct. A child's primary attitudes about sexuality are formed before the age of five, whether these have come actively and positively from caring parents or whether they have come from neighborhood peers or from hours in front of the television. Parents are the primary sex educators of their children all during the pre-school years. This teaching takes place when parents bathe their child, react to a bowel movement, or cuddle their youngster. It is their expressions of simple warmth, calm acceptance, and total trust that pave the way to healthy, responsible, loving, and caring attitudes about a person's sexuality. Parents need to be much more involved in their children's sexual learning in the early years, before their children enter school.

MYTH 2: *Very few children name their parents as their first choice for sexual information.*

Survey after survey tell us that most children prefer to hear about sex from their parents first. That's the good news. Unfortunately, when most of the information is given by them it is not at the right time or is incomplete or untrue. Many parents become embarrassed and flustered by the language of sexuality. People who consistently confuse discussions of sexuality by boasting or telling jokes are only trying to hide their own insecurity. Children are very sensitive about the emotional value that parents give to certain words. If you are severely inhibited when talking about sex, you more than likely cannot transmit healthy attitudes to your children. Rather than have our children turn to other sources for information we do not agree with, like their peers or television, let's take our responsibility and be prepared to meet their questions with good information and intelligent conversation.

MYTH 3: *Sex education in the home is primarily the responsibility of the parent of the same sex.*

Sex education is properly the responsibility of *both* parents, for both boys and girls, as it is reflected in their relationship and in communication with their children. The days of the one session father/son or mother/daughter talk are gone. They were never very helpful. Children like to learn attitudes and values from both parents, so they need honest and open facts about males and females from both their mothers and their fathers. Some fathers, unfortunately, fail to realize the importance of their contribution and simply refuse to say anything about sex to their children. This is too often the norm in most homes. If your husband refuses to take part in his children's education, you must take it upon yourself to explain love, God and sex to all your children. Incidentally, it has never been established that girls are better educated by their mothers or boys by their fathers. Single parents can relax and do a fine job.

MYTH 4: *Today's young people already know everything there is to know about sex.*

Where did they learn it? What attitudes and values came with it? Who taught them this information, and is it accurate? Our children need the facts, clear and scientifically correct, and encouragement to support the value systems we ourselves came to know and cherish in our own relationships. Ironically, sexually experienced young people often feel compelled to exaggerate their knowledge, to pretend they understand as much as their experience suggests. In 1977 a Johns Hopkins University study of 15–17 year old girls found that only thrity-seven percent knew when in the menstrual cycle the risk of conception was greatest, and it was clear that most of them were having intercourse exactly at that time. Younger children require information to be repeated several times until a complete, well-rounded understanding can be absorbed.

MYTH 5: *Parents have to know a lot to be able to teach their children about sexuality.*

Parents only need to be willing to say, "We'll look it up." Your children don't expect you to be experts in the field. But they do need you to be askable. Once the question has been asked and the parent has accepted it without fear, then half the work is done. Facts can be found in any library. Loving, compassionate, sensitive parents are only found within themselves.

MYTH 6: *You can harm children by telling them "too much."*

The worst this will do is bore them. A little information that is "over their heads" simply sets the stage for your next talk. Children are more interested that you've shown your willingness to be open than that you have miscalculated exactly how much they were ready to comprehend. Rest assured, no one advocates pumping three or four year olds with great quantities of information about pregnancy or intercourse. We simply want to assure well-intentioned parents that they will not harm their children by *answering* questions, only by refusing to tell the truth to them.

MYTH 7: *It is always best to wait until a child asks.*

"When should I tell?" The answer is simple: as early as possible, and certainly whenever the child asks or shows interest in other ways. Your children may begin to ask sex questions from the time they are two. With young children, the questions are sometimes non-verbal. For example, a child may constantly follow you into the bathroom. Some shy children might ask no questions at all. If your child hasn't raised sexual questions by the age of four, don't wait, but start the conversation. There are many daily situations that can be used as conversation starters. For children who read, leave a book out in a convenient spot. Television programs sometimes provide a lead into a discussion on a specific sexual issue. Tell them about a neighbor or a relative who is going to have a baby. Make sure they hear from you that sex and love go together.

MYTH 8: *Most parents are opposed to sex education programs offered in schools.*

Surveys indicate that over eighty-three percent of parents *approve* of schools giving courses in sex education to their children. Most parents are also primarily and properly concerned about what values will be taught along with the facts. The successful sex education program will have the support and participation of teachers, parents, administrators, and the community. The best programs emphasize helping students build a system of values to guide their behavior in making decisions about all relationships, including sexual ones. Such a program provides students not only with facts, but with opportunities to test attitudes and beliefs learned from the home with the teacher and fellow students. The primary advantage in a Church-sponsored school is that the values taught will be consistent with and supportive of the family beliefs initiated in the home. We need to realize that there are some things no school can or should try to provide. For example, the school will not relieve parents of their responsibility for helping build values, especially when a person is attending a Church-sponsored school whose teachings are consistent with the family's moral tradition. A good school program will neither lessen sexual promiscuity nor increase it through the stimulation of natural curiosity. It will serve to help to reduce venereal disease, eliminate unwanted pregnancies and prevent ill-advised marriages.

Sex education should seek to provide young people with the skills, knowledge and attitudes that will enable them to make decisions based on the values and beliefs they respect and trust for daily living. As parents, we need to be reassured that our standards of family living and values will be supported. We are the most influential sex educators of our children as long as we accept and act on that responsibility and realize that any school program is only supplementary.

MYTH 9: *Increasingly, professionals and parents agree that programs in sex education should be exclusively taught to teenagers.*

Our focus in sexual learning is that it is a lifelong process, not confined to the teen period. Since fundamental attitudes about sex are formed at a very early age, it is important that parents begin teaching their children from birth. This does not mean that the factual content should be the same for young children as for teens. Rather, simple, clear and correct facts given with the family's value framework to young children will, if continued and enlarged throughout childhood, ensure their future emotional and spiritual health as it relates to their sexuality.

MYTH 10: *Parents who do not talk about sex with their younger children will be unable to influence their teenagers later in life.*

This situation is most common in many homes today. However, a parent might begin a conversation with their teenager in this way: "I really made a mistake by waiting this long, and I wish we had talked when you were younger. Now I understand why you might feel embarrassed to talk with me." Plan ahead for such discussions. Have a book ready. Tell your child that you think he or she might be interested in it. Explain that some of the material need not embarrass him or her, and that you're going to leave the book around to start the discussion rolling. The main thing for him or her to understand is that you are available to talk whenever he or she is ready.

MYTH 11: *Sex education causes more unwed pregnancies.*

Many parents fear that sex education causes sexual experimentation and promiscuity, resulting in increased numbers of teenage pregnancies. This is definitely not true. Surveys indicate that people who have taken a sex education course do not change the frequency or the way they express their sexual behavior, nor do they become more liberal in their attitudes. They do appear to become more accepting of others' differing attitudes and behavior. However, when contraception information is included in the curriculum, such courses help students to become more effective users of family planning methods, and this can help to reduce the number of teenage pregnancies.

MYTH: 12: *Training programs fail significantly to help parents talk with their children about sex.*

Before there can be sex education for children, there must first be sex education for parents who may never have had any. Evidence has proved that programs designed to help parents become knowledgeable, more open and more relaxed in talking about sex provide the best atmosphere for parent-child communication. Parents need to be encouraged to take the lead in becoming more comfortable in dealing with their children's sexual questions. There is no reason why a father shouldn't answer some of his daughter's questions. Also, a mother can talk with her son as well as she can with her daughter. In one-parent families, this is the way it has to be handled. If both parents are equally prepared, questions can be dealt with as they occur and answered by whichever parent happens to be present. And the child knows that the parents share the same knowledge and values.

Many church communities strongly endorse programs in sex education which prepare parents to serve as the primary sex educators of their children. Besides contributing information and helping parents to be frank and open, the Church provides an atmosphere for learning and reflecting on religious attitudes and values unique to each religious tradition. Within the Catholic community and other traditions, there is an urgent, serious invitation to begin this work. We encourage you to help to develop and share this model program with other interested parents to further develop programs in your church community.

> MYTH 13: *Children who see their parents in sexual intercourse suffer from harmful effects later in life.*

People hold differing attitudes about children's presence during their parents' love making. Certainly infants below the age of about a year have some awareness but little comprehension of actions that are not directed at themselves. As children grow their awareness increases much faster than their understanding. Quite young children may be aware of the physical actions of their parents. If so, they may interpret actions of foreplay and intercourse as "fighting" or other violence.

Most specialists in child studies recommend that children not share their parents' bedroom. Both the parents and children need some undisturbed privacy. However, if a child does walk in on his parents during intercourse, the effect on the child depends primarily on the parents' reaction. If parents react with horror and scolding, the child will remember the incident with guilt and fear. If parents remain calm, reassure the child that they are not fighting or hurting each other, and remind the child that closed doors mean that people want to have some private time, there should be no harmful effects on the child.

Children should not have routine casual access to adults having intercourse. This is a private, personal, adult activity that children are not fully capable of dealing with. But the accidental encounter, common to many homes, is seldom harmful.

Physiological

> MYTH 14: *Nocturnal emissions, "wet dreams," indicate an abnormal sexual behavior.*

Wet dreams are perfectly normal and quite common among adolescents and adults. They serve a useful purpose of lowering sexual tension. Neither is this behavior restricted to men. Women have similar dreams and physical arousal, even to climax, although they do not ejaculate as males do. There is nothing shameful or abnormal about the male wet dream. There is no value for any child in being shocked or startled by these experiences. Children should be prepared to recognize them as normal aspects of sexual development that also mark the beginning of the male's capacity to father a child.

MYTH 15: *Penis or breast size increases a person's sexual pleasure and performance.*

Men and women are often concerned about genital size because in our society we have come to equate bigger with better. The size of a man's penis or a woman's breasts has nothing to do with sexual pleasure or performance. Time or energy spent worrying about these is wasted. Many people mistakenly equate a large penis with greater masculinity. Flaccid penis size varies considerably from male to male. There is little relationship between the size of a flaccid penis and its size when erect. And there is less relationship between penile and general body size than exists between the dimensions of the other organs and the body. Furthermore, breast size in no way affects the ability to breast feed. Any healthy woman can successfully nurse her infant.

MYTH 16: *Masturbation is a habit of the young and immature; its practice typically ceases after marriage.*

Masturbation means to touch one's own sex organs in a way that brings pleasure, usually to experience orgasm. Masturbation is common throughout infancy, childhood and adolescence and among people of all ages because it brings comfort and a release of tension. It is a way of getting to know one's body intimately. Masturbation has been the subject of all sorts of myths; that it was mentally unhealthy, the cause of blindness, acne and other physical deformities and even insanity. None of these myths are true.

The teaching of the Catholic Church originally focused its attention on the physical behavior; masturbation was unnatural because a man who masturbated ejaculated sperm without the intention of intercourse. The teaching today focuses less on the biological dimension of this behavior. Rather, it is seen as a wrong use of the sexual organs because sexual expression ideally should take place in the context of a loving relationship with one's married spouse.

MYTH 17: *Many teenagers know all about their fertility cycle and just when the risk of pregnancy is greatest.*

The shocking evidence reveals that most young people are ignorant of their fertility. Twelve, thirteen, and fourteen year old children have sexual intercourse. In addition, the earlier their age, the less they usually know about it. Parents are shocked to think that their children are involved in sexual experimentation. Whether anyone likes it or not, more than half of all high school students will have had sexual intercourse before graduation. We are opposed to teenagers having sexual intercourse. We need to tell our young people that they are too young, too vulnerable. The double standard is still very much with us. Boys still use such lines as, "If you really love me, you'll have sex with me." Girls rarely reply with, "If you really loved me, you wouldn't put this pressure on me." In addition, teenage pregnancy is unsound from the medical, moral, and psychological points of view.

Parents must face the possibility that however clear they have made their own values, their teenagers may just as clearly reject them. Should this occur, however, parents can still exert a positive influence. Without anger and without condemnation, parents can simply say, "We do not want you to have intercourse, but if your mind is already made up, at least become aware of how to avoid pregnancy." It is important to realize that providing information about fertility does not mean that young people will be more promiscuous. Rather than risk teenagers having children, some people decide to use contraception. This means that they prevent sperm from reaching the egg and fertilizing it or they prevent the egg from being released into the fallopian tubes. As Catholic parents, this issue causes confusion, guilt, and frustration. There are many ways to practice birth control; in fact, technology is constantly providing new methods. However, we know that not all have the official approval of the Catholic Church. This is the struggle and challenge which faces our Catholic couples today. It is the topic about which many women feel anger, bitterness, and resentment for the Church's lack of understanding. Let's try to offer some truth and compassion about this issue, especially when talking to our teenagers.

First, it is our duty to explain birth control to our teenagers. Silence about this topic is irresponsible, and an abomination to the Gospel message that says we are to be honest and compassionate in our relationships with others. Some messages that we need to make clear to our young people are that abstinence is always one hundred percent effective. It's all right not to have sex. *Not* everyone is having intercourse. In the past many couples refrained from intercourse around the time the woman was supposed to be fertile. This method was called rhythm and was approved by the Church. Today this method is no longer accepted because a woman is not always regular enough in her biological cycle.

A more dependable method which is approved by the Church is called the symptomo-thermal method, or "natural family planning." This method determines through natural means when a woman will be fertile. It requires instruction to help the man and woman appreciate and understand the woman's fertility based on her regular menstrual cycle. The couple learns to determine the time of fertility by charting her menstrual cycle, paying close attention to her body temperature and mucous discharge. At first there is a period of abstinence which the couple needs to practice. Many couples who successfully use this method claim that it helps their relationship to grow. There are many "natural family planning" agencies in dioceses which provide initial and follow-up instruction to help couples practice this method correctly.

Other methods of birth control lack Church approval because they interfere artificially with the possibility of the sperm fertilizing the egg. Some methods, like foams, or the new sponge/foam method, kill the sperm with chemicals placed in the vagina. A diaphragm blocks the entrance to the uterus, and "condoms" cover the penis with rubber to prevent sperm from entering the vagina, while they help to prevent the spread of venereal disease. Intrauterine devices, or IUD's, alter the lining of the woman's uterus so that the egg will not attach itself. The "pill" prevents the egg from being released, or may prevent implantation.

Surgical procedures that prevent pregnancy are referred to as sterilization. In a man who has a vasectomy, the tubes through which the sperm travel are cut. A woman can have her fallopian tubes cut and tied so that sperm cannot reach the eggs to fertilize them. These are generally permanent methods of birth control.

The Catholic Church traditionally has held the position that these forms of preventing conception are wrong because they do not leave the act of intercourse open to the possibility of creating new life. Most people disagree with this teaching. Many Catholic parents use medical birth control for the sake of their marriage, knowing that these methods are more effective than the biological methods. While many couples who have made this decision have disregarded the Church's teaching, others have reflected on it and decided to follow it. An important fact is that many women are not regular or not comfortable enough with their bodies in their biological cycle or in their life style to determine through natural means when they are fertile.

What are the messages we want to get across to our young people about this unsettling issue? First, we are opposed to teenagers having intercourse. Second, beyond avoiding conception, are they aware of the possible consequences of using birth control? Some methods can have a harmful effect on the body in some people. Third, how will the use of birth control affect the relationship with the partner? Fourth, will your decision about birth control affect your response to the message of Jesus? Couples who ponder these questions with the help of a compassionate spiritual advisor may reach different conclusions. Whatever decision is reached, it's important that the couple take responsibility for their sexual relationship. Finally, we need to say to our young people that whatever choice they make, the Church, while not necessarily agreeing with it, must still accept and love them. Shame, rejection and fear are not the ways of God. Rather, trust in God's judgment is the basic message we want to give to our young people.

MYTH 18: *It is harmful to have intercourse while menstruating.*

Intercourse during menstruation is a matter of preference. There is no indication that this causes any harmful side-effects. Many women report heightened sexual receptivity before and during their periods.

MYTH 19: *Only girls need to know that when they experience their first menstrual period, they can become pregnant.*

Both boys and girls need to understand menstruation in girls and ejaculation in boys. There is no excuse for any child to arrive unprepared at these points in life. The appearance of the first menstrual flow generally indicates that a girl will soon produce a mature ovum (egg) which is ready to be fertilized, although rarely a girl will become pregnant before she has ever menstruated. However, young people always need to hear the message that pregnancy before the age of eighteen is not a good idea for any woman. Also, intercourse is not necessary in order to be happy or healthy. Teenagers are physically, emotionally, and spiritually unprepared for parenthood.

MYTH 20: *In most cases, married couples are unable to conceive a child because the female is infertile.*

Statistics show that about fifty percent of all failure to conceive is the result of male infertility. However, in most male-dominated societies like ours, the wife is often, unfortunately, made to feel guilty for failing to fulfill her role as a mother. This situation is false and unnecessary and leads to unhappiness and frustration.

Medical examination for infertility is necessary after an unsuccessful conception effort of six to nine months in women under thirty and one year in women over thirty years of age. It is necessary for the couple to go to a physician together. No woman should undergo any infertility workup unless her partner is also examined by a urologist or gynecologist knowledgeable in the field of male fertility and given a clean bill of health regarding sperm count, motility, and cellular structure. This is simply because a man need only provide a sperm sample, whereas a woman's evaluation is expensive and time-consuming and can be unpleasant.

Unfortunately, many men refuse this rather simple examination for fear of being found deficient in sperm, an ego-shattering prospect for an insecure man. Education, explanation, medication, and compassion can help a man in this situation.

MYTH 21: *Once a male becomes sexually excited to the point of having an erection, it is physically harmful for him to refrain from sexual intercourse.*

This attitude is a "line" men frequently use in attempting to persuade their partners to have intercourse. It is untrue and expresses attitudes of manipulation and dishonesty which prevent responsible, caring relationships from developing. Although prolonged sexual excitation for a male may lead to a painful aching in the genital area, this condition is not physiologically harmful and will ultimately subside in the absence of further sexual stimulation.

MYTH 22: *The penis must ejaculate in the vagina for pregnancy to occur.*

Impregnation is possible without penetration and it happens quite often. If the penis is near or on the labia when ejaculation occurs, sperm can enter the vaginal opening and make their way to the uterus.

In addition, the pre-ejaculation fluid often contains enough sperm to make their way to the uterus and cause pregnancy even though the man's penis has never entered the vagina.

MYTH 23: *A woman's sexual desires disappear after menopause.*

Survey after survey has shown that whatever a woman's sexual capacity has been previously, it usually continues undiminished until into her sixties or older. This is long past the age of menopause for most women. A woman's sex drive does not diminish if she loses her ovaries or their hormone production. Hormones are only one of the many factors affecting capacity for sexual response. A more important factor is the woman's attitude toward sex.

MYTH 24: *Only women fake orgasm.*

It is true that many women do this all their lives, and their spouses may never know it. However, this attitude can be very degrading to women when it implies that it is only women who fake orgasm. The implication is that males always experience orgasm when they have intercourse. This is not true. A person's pleasure in orgasm is quite variable. It is important to stress the need for open and honest communication about sexual matters within marriage. Equality in sexual satisfaction seems desirable and can be best achieved through open sharing of desires and concerns.

MYTH 25: *A woman has a lower sex drive than a man and/or her sexual needs are less important.*

Current evidence indicates that women have at least the same degree of sexual desire as men. This issue can be the source of great hurt and anxiety for many women later in life. What we want to stress is the equality of their right to sexual fulfillment for all persons. We have to convey to our young people that the biased, prejudiced attitude that "wives should always be submissive" to the dominant male was never the intention of the biblical writer. Rather, males who use this "line" to obtain sex are exploiting the passage for their own selfish purposes. The message to get across is the responsibility that couples have to make each other feel accepted, cared for, and appreciated. A relationship based on this foundation generates equality and mutual respect and concern for a spouse's sexual needs.

MYTH 26: *Simultaneous orgasms are necessary for pregnancy to occur.*

The myth of mutual orgasm being necessary for pregnancy to occur is widespread. There is no organ in the female or male that must be triggered by the female's orgasm before pregnancy can occur. In fact, women who have never experienced orgasm can and do conceive.

MYTH 27: *Pre-menstrual syndrome (PMS) is part of being a woman which has no physical cause.*

Pre-menstrual syndrome is the term which refers to a wide variety of physical and psychological symptoms that women can experience one to ten days before their period begins. Studies have found that PMS most likely results from an imbalance in the production of hormones which control the menstrual cycle. Many women who experience discomfort from PMS have either too little progesterone (the hormone that stimulates the thickening of the uterine lining) or too much estrogen in relation to progesterone. Evidence which points to a hormonal imbalance is that PMS only occurs on those days when progesterone should be present at a high level. After menstruation, when progesterone is not produced by the body, the symptoms of PMS never occur.

A wide variety of physical and psychological symptoms have been identified. Physical symptoms include: water retention, tender breasts, food cravings, headaches, migraines, aches and pains, clumsiness, and fatigue. Some of the psychological symptoms include: tension, anxiety, irritability, depression, lethargy, and insomnia. A holistic approach to health recognizes the intertwining of physical and psychological events. For example, if a woman's body retains extra water before her period, she may put on weight and feel bloated. This can make her feel depressed and lethargic—an example of the physical leading to the psychological. Or feelings of tension and anxiety can produce headaches or migraines—the psychological leading to the physical.

Once a woman is aware that she suffers from PMS, she can begin to do something about it. Being careful about proper diet, reducing stress, and getting proper exercise can provide some relief. If these don't provide sufficient comfort, a woman may find medical help. Women have been ridiculed about PMS for too long, and there are many things women can do for themselves. Most important, PMS should never be taken as an excuse to deny women opportunities in ministry or at work.

MYTH 28: *Alcohol is a sexual stimulant.*

The truth is that alcohol is a depressant. It retards reflexes and dilates blood vessels; thus, among other things, it interferes with the capacity for erection in males and increases genital engorgement in females. Alcohol does temporarily relieve feelings of sexual guilt and fear as a by-product of depressing the inhibition mechanisms of the brain. So with only one or two drinks, alcohol as a physical depressant and as a factor lessening inhibitions probably balances out. However, getting past the stresses of the moment through good communication or resolving the emotional conflicts concerning sexuality would probably do more for sexual functioning than would alcohol.

General Health

MYTH 29: *Regular douching is necessary to keep the vagina clean.*

Most douching is not only unnecessary, because the natural secretions of a healthy woman keep her vaginal tract clean, but it is considered undesirable by most competent gynecologists. In fact, frequent douching can be harmful by destroying the beneficial organisms of the vagina or by masking symptoms of some conditions that may need medical attention. Douching has no effectiveness as a means of contraception. Young girls should be helped to be proud that they possess such a wonderful, unique, self-cleaning organ as the vagina. They should be taught to wash their hands, which may be dirty, before they touch themselves in dressing or bathing.

MYTH 30: *A woman does not need a Pap smear test until she has had a child or reached middle age.*

A Pap smear is a procedure that detects the earliest stage of cervical cancer, which is one of the most common malignancies found in women. It can be readily detected with a high degree of accuracy. Pre-cancerous conditions (severe dysplasia) and localized early cancer (carcinoma in situ) can be diagnosed and properly treated before serious problems occur.

The Pap smear is a screening procedure and tells the physician which patients need further investigation. The smear is obtained by taking a small wooden spatula and gently scraping the opening to the cervix, no more painful than scratching the inside of your mouth with your fingernail. The material obtained from cervical secretions is spread on a glass slide and sent to a laboratory for microscopic examination to detect vaginitis, venereal disease, or other possible infections. The procedure is painless, and the American Cancer Society recommends that it should be performed on all women at least once a year beginning at the age of twenty.

During the pelvic examination, in addition to making a visual and manual examination, the doctor draws blood samples to be tested for syphilis, sugar level, blood counts, blood type, RH factor, and possibly other factors. Urine is collected for complete microscopic examination to discover any abnormal cells or abnormal components such as sugar and albumin.

MYTH 31: *Fetal alcohol syndrome (FAS) is a minor problem for pregnant women that can be prevented by consuming alcohol in moderation.*

Fetal alcohol syndrome is a real problem for more than one million alcoholic women of child-bearing age. FAS is a real tragedy because it is totally preventable and because the damage to the infant is irreversible. Everything the pregnant woman eats or drinks passes freely through the placenta to her baby. The alcohol that the baby gets is as strong as that which the mother takes. Studies show that alcohol consumed by the expectant mother remains in the blood of the baby twice as long as it does in her own. During pregnancy, alcohol affects the baby's rapidly growing tissue, either killing cells or slowing their growth. The brain is the organ most in jeopardy. One common symptom of FAS is growth deficiency.

Affected babies are abnormally small at birth, especially in head size. Unlike many small newborns, however, FAS babies never catch up to normal growth. Small brains accompanied by mild to moderate mental retardation are characteristic. Evidence today shows that their IQ's do not improve with age. Almost half have heart defects.

No one knows how little—or how much—alcohol may damage an unborn baby. Initially, FAS was thought to affect only the children of chronic, habitual drinkers. Researchers now believe that sporadic exposure to concentrated amounts of alcohol (binge drinking) may be equally dangerous. Other studies suggest that even moderate drinking is associated with retarded fetal growth.

Given these facts, the March of Dimes now recommends complete abstinence from alcohol during pregnancy, since no safe level of alcohol consumption and no safe time during the pregnancy have been determined. One of the most frightening aspects of FAS is that the damage can occur as early as the third week after conception, well before most women even suspect they are pregnant.

MYTH 32: *Teenage pregnancy and childbirth are not severe health risks.*

Numerous studies conducted during the last few years have indicated that many teenagers are sexually active and that their sexual activity has produced severe problems both for them and for society. Each year, approximately 1.3 million girls between the ages of ten and nineteen become pregnant. About 700,000 of these will miscarry or have abortions. On the average, each day about 3,300 girls become pregnant. More than one-third of all adolescent girls become pregnant before they are twenty years old. Overall, the consequences of these teenage pregnancies are tragic. The main cause for the higher health risk in women under eighteen is that the typical unmarried, pregnant teenager in our society does not, for a number of reasons, receive the medical attention, nutritional advice, and general support equivalent to those given a typical married pregnant women. Many unmarried, pregnant teenage

girls hide their pregnancies for too long, and, as a result, both they and their babies suffer. The 600,000 babies actually born to teenagers each year show more deaths, health problems, pre-maturity, and mental retardation than do babies born to women over eighteen. Teenage mothers much less often finish school than do the unmarried over eighteen, and both they and the young men involved suffer the economic consequences of reduced education for the rest of their lives. Teenage mothers are also far more likely than other teenagers to become dependent upon welfare and remain on it for life. Some teenage mothers decide to marry the men involved, but such marriages almost always end in divorce. Each year several hundred thousand adolescents choose to terminate their pregnancies through abortion. For some, these abortions have serious physical, emotional, and social consequences.

The Catholic Church teaches that abortion is wrong because it destroys innocent human life. Since 1973, when a Supreme Court ruling overturned most of the laws that prohibited abortion in this country, the Church has been joined by other voices. Many groups have formed to present the "Pro Life" view that human life should not be destroyed, even in the womb, for the convenience of another person.

Abortion is not new. For thousands of years women have been terminating unwanted pregnancies with herbs, poisons, or wires inserted into their bodies because they were so desperate; they were actually risking their lives in order to get rid of the unwanted babies within them. Unscrupulous people would take advantage of their desperation, charge high fees for abortions and then perform them under unsanitary conditions. Such women often died.

No one wants to see women return to this desperate state. Fortunately, society today is more open to the idea that women may bear children out of wedlock. They are no longer publicly denounced. No one wants to see women die in childbirth or have their health permanently scarred because of a complicated pregnancy either, but life and death abortions are a small percentage of the millions that have been performed in this country since 1973.

People who advocate keeping abortion legal call their outlook "Pro Choice." They believe that it is up to the woman to decide whether to continue a pregnancy. They fear that laws against abortion will bring back the days when women would risk life and health to have one. They believe that the woman's right to control her body is more important than the unborn child. There are many sincere people who feel this way, including some Catholics.

It is important to make a distinction between a person's opinion and the person. It's always a temptation to condemn people who hold a different view, but this is not Jesus' way. Judgment is reserved for the Lord. What is important is taking responsibility for our own opinions and actions. If we oppose abortion, it follows that we must also make a commitment to care for the children who will be born to women who otherwise might have had the abortions.

There are a number of agencies that can help teenagers and their families cope. A parish priest can make referrals to a Catholic social service agency. Birthright is another agency that can help you decide. We should realize that this is a complex issue that demands our sensitivity and compassion when talking with young people who face this crisis.

MYTH 33: *Contraceptive education results in increased sexual activity among teenagers.*

A 1982 study found that a sex education course does not result in increased sexual activity among unmarried young men and women. But it also showed that sexually active young women who took sex education courses which included information on birth control methods are more likely to use contraceptives and are less likely to become pregnant than those who had no such instruction. (Results of a comparative study of two high schools, by Johns Hopkins University professors Melvin Zelnik and Young J. Kim, reported in the May/June 1982 issue of *Family Planning Perspectives*.)

Many people believe that the primary responsibility for family planning and for decisions about contraception and what method to use is the woman's. This is wrong. The most successful users of family planning are those couples who decide together what method to use and who practice it together. The message that parents must explain to their teenagers

41

is: "We really think you're much too young to have sex, but if you're not going to listen to us, know something about birth control. More important, we don't ever want you to feel that there is anything you can't talk to us about."

MYTH 34: *Venereal disease is not a major problem for teenagers.*

Tragically, surveys indicate that increased teenage sexual activity has brought them widespread infection. In 1983 the Center for Disease Control reported that 228,000 young people between the ages of ten and nineteen contracted a venereal disease. As responsible parents, we must provide teenagers with information and encourage them to practice prevention. The fact we want to convey is that venereal diseases are spread by sexual contact. They can be transmitted by an infected person any time that he or she has sexual contact—homosexual or heterosexual—or mouth-to-genital contact. It is not necessary to have an orgasm or even to enjoy the sex act to contract VD. VD germs live only in warm, moist areas like the genitals, the mouth, or the rectum. Air and dryness will kill them; therefore, they cannot be picked up from toilet seats or doorknobs, although they can be spread, in rare instances, by kissing. Venereal disease is now more accurately referred to as sexually transmitted disease (STD). The most dangerous types of sexually transmitted diseases are herpes, gonorrhea, syphilis, and a new disease called AIDS (acquired immune deficiency syndrome). Gonorrhea is now the second most communicable disease in our nation—second only to the common cold. Herpes genitalis is now the second most common sexually transmitted disease, surpassed in frequency only by gonorrhea.

Gonorrhea and syphilis can be cured quickly—usually with penicillin therapy or antibiotics—if treated in the early stages. A teenager does not need parental consent, or even knowledge, for diagnosis and treatment, even if he or she is a minor. Therefore, a person should go immediately to a VD clinic, health center or private doctor if VD is suspected. VD centers test for VD without charge and do not inform the parents, but will provide free treatment and contact the sexual partners of the infected persons. Self-treatment is almost always useless. Treating sores with a penicillin ointment often kills only the top layers and leaves the germs underneath alive and spreading.

We realize that the infected person suffers the additional pain of guilt, shame, and embarrassment. All the moralizing in the world won't heal this epidemic unless we encourage our teenagers by being willing to help and have prepared ourselves to do so. We must educate ourselves with information regarding detection, prevention, the importance of early treatment, and where to go for treatment. If we continue to pass on attitudes of embarrassment and condemnation toward syphilis and gonorrhea and herpes, these venereal diseases will continue to spread among our young people. Compassion, accurate information, and support for VD programs can help to break the conspiracy of silence and fear that surrounds the disease and prevent the danger to many young people.

MYTH 35: *AIDS is a plague sent by God to punish homosexuals.*

AIDS (Acquired Immune Deficiency Syndrome) is a complex disease. Due to its newness and seriousness, much research is being done and new information will probably be available by the time this book is printed. According to current understanding, AIDS is caused by an infectious agent, most probably a virus, which attacks the immune or germ-fighting system of a person. The person is then susceptible to many diseases that people with normal immune systems are seldom troubled by. AIDS is believed to be transmitted by contact with blood or blood fluids of an infected person. Anal or oral-anal intercourse, use of shared needles for drug injection and contaminated blood products are most commonly suspected. Normal daily household contact and contact in the delivery of health care have *not* been realized as ways of transmitting AIDS.

The most common victims seem to be homosexual men (frequent anal intercourse), intravenous drug users (contaminated needles), hemophiliacs (concentrated blood products from many donors), and Haitians (for unknown reasons).

The AIDS problem has produced understandable concern within the homosexual community. But the fear and animosity toward gays as a group by others is completely unfounded. In the past few decades, medical science has seen the outbreak of several diseases that were previously unknown.

MYTH 36: *Toxic shock syndrome (TSS) is a common and fatal disease associated with tampon use in menstruating girls and women.*

Toxic shock syndrome is believed to be caused by a toxin released by the bacterium, Staphylococcus Aureus. It is found in the vagina of about two to fifteen percent of all women. It is almost one hundred percent present in TSS cases, and the strain of bacterium seems to be penicillin resistant. Several theories as to why tampons are associated with the disease have been proposed; none have, as yet, been substantiated. As many as fifteen of every 100,000 menstruating girls and women will get the disease each year. TSS is a rare disease. Publicity has helped us become aware of its symptoms such as fever (102°F or greater), headache, sore throat, vomiting or diarrhea, muscle aches, rash that looks like sunburn, and peeling of skin on palms and soles.

Menstruating women are not the only ones at risk. TSS has been diagnosed in males and young children. The low risk of TSS in women is almost entirely eliminated if sanitary pads are used instead of tampons. Girls and women who choose to use tampons will minimize the risk if they use tampons intermittently during their period (i.e., use pads at night, change tampons at least every eight hours, wash their hands before inserting a tampon and insert the tampon carefully to avoid carrying bacteria into the vagina). If a woman has been diagnosed as having TSS, or if she suspects she has had it, she should not use tampons until her doctor advises her that it is all right to do so.

Marriage and Family Life

MYTH 37: *Adolescents who mature physically earlier become sexually active earlier.*

A mature physical appearance does not necessarily indicate emotional readiness for sexual activity. Adolescents who mature physically ahead of their peers may feel self-conscious about how different they and their friends are, and this may pressure them to social activities with an older group. Open and frank discussion of these pressures can help them decide how and with whom they want to spend their time.

MYTH 38: *Marriage is the most acceptable solution for pregnant teenagers.*

Tragically, in cases of unwed pregnancy, parents of teenagers often think more of their own embarrassment than of their children's welfare. In a few cases where the young people love each other and are ready for this responsibility, this may be the best choice. However, many parents believe that every pregnancy must be covered up by a wedding which pushes couples to the altar in fear rather than love. Perhaps the strongest first impulse of a Christian is to cover the sin. Society and the teachings of the Church used to attach a lifelong stigma to an illegitimate child. The problem is that if a couple is not prepared for marriage, their embarrassment has barely begun.

Family and friends get a sense of reassurance, but the young people get a lifetime commitment they neither wanted nor were ready for. Though parents may feel that the sin of premarital sex has been covered, in fact we have merely added something more sinful: professing Christian marriage on a false basis. We need to share with our children a vision of marriage that goes beyond bringing life into the world, but includes nurturing fidelity, friendship, and intimacy in a lifelong, loving relationship.

MYTH 39: *Couples who choose not to marry after having conceived a child convey their lack of faithfulness to the "marriage" they made when they went to bed.*

If we accept this attitude, we are going to have to change many of our basic principles in the Christian faith. The purpose of the sacrament of marriage is found in God's love for his people and the couple's desire to imitate that love before God, their families, and the Christian community. There is no such finality with two people who, engrossed in passion or curiosity, go to bed with each other. Sex does not make a marriage. Sex is an important part of marriage. It leads to growth and acceptance of persons who strive to be lovers, friends, and partners for a lifetime. However, marriage should take place not with overheated bodies, but with clear, binding promises.

MYTH 40: *Many teenagers use marriage as an opportunity for unlimited sexual activity.*

The message parents should convey is that they are opposed to teenagers having intercourse for which they are not ready. They are too vulnerable for exploitation. Also, marriage is not a license that gives people the right to abuse or exploit a spouse. Some young people mistakenly think of marriage as the only way to express their sexuality. This is not true. Young people need to know that sexuality is concerned with issues besides intercourse, pregnancy, and birth control. Knowing about mature love, which generates healthy friendships, is of great importance to young people. Helping teenagers feel good about themselves and developing their interest in life helps them develop enjoyable relationships. Mature relationships are difficult for people who feel inferior or inadequate. Marriage in itself is no cure for pervasive feelings of inferiority. On the contrary, such feelings work against a successful marriage.

MYTH 41: *Only a person who marries can be a sexual person.*

Children are sexual the moment they are conceived. Their sexuality is never dependent on the lifestyle they choose later in life. Rather, the parts of their lives that make them male or female, all their experiences, their relationships, their learnings, and their knowledge, make them sexual beings. They are gifted with a sexual nature. As they grow, they need to learn how best to use this gift to bring joy, care and happiness into all their relationships. Sexual relationships need not and most often do not involve genital sex. People, whether living as married couples, single parents, celibates, heterosexuals, or homosexuals, are all sexual people in the sense that they all relate to each other as a female or male at each given moment in all of their relationships.

MYTH 42: *As persons grow older, they generally lose interest in sexual activity and their sexual drive decreases.*

Sexuality plays a significant role in all our relationships at all stages of life. There is no evidence to support the idea that as one grows older, his or her sense of sexuality diminishes. Often the real issue which concerns the elderly is the lack of encouragement and opportunity to express their sexuality. The younger generation's shock and embarrassment only contributes to handicapping a normal, healthy condition in life. It also breeds the double standard, which degrades all of human life. The message we should convey is that we were created for close, warm bodily and emotional contact. The essence of our created natures was emphasized as being "very good." That includes our sexuality which we discover at every stage of our lives. It does not have to diminish nor should we feel ashamed about it with the coming of age.

Particular Issues

MYTH 43: *Sex education is unimportant for persons with disabilities.*

Disabled young people need special messages that say their sexual needs or desires are blessed, healthy, and normal. Children from whom sexual information is kept secret, who are discouraged from asking questions, scolded for experimentation, shamed for being found out, and denied both the privacy and the social opportunities to explore their natural sexuality, will probably suffer more than normal adolescents under the same circumstances. To deny the sexuality of handicapped youth is to oppress them further. It is not a kindness to structure their lives so as to close off the entire area of sexuality; it is handicapping them a second time and denying them their God-given birthright.

We strongly encourage people who work with disabled children and adolescents to include in their treatment programs information and skills that will encourage them to accept responsibility for their lives and their sexual activities. Their true need is for the accurate knowledge, which is their best protection, and for as much freedom and independence as their impairment permits. The disabled must be taught about love, caring, marriage, conception, birth, contraception, and venereal disease.

The main problem that many people with disabilities have is that they have been made to feel inferior. One of the primary messages we can give is that no one can make you feel inferior without your consent. At a meeting with several hundred severely handicapped people, with their parents and teachers present, a comment was made by a workshop participant who was responsible for a group of severely cerebral palsied adults in wheelchairs. She stated, "How can anyone claim these people don't feel inferior when they only need to look at themselves in a mirror to know that message represents empty promises of a future that is not possible for any of them?" The right response came from a beautiful woman confined to a wheelchair. She said, "You know, when I look at myself I feel depressed. When I take in the world I live in, I'm impressed. And when I allow God to touch me, I feel blessed." This response pointed to a group of people wanting desperately to talk about their hidden aspirations, their desire for love, companionship, and sexual expression. There are very few limitations that people with disabilities, their parents, their teachers, and all of us with them cannot overcome.

MYTH 44: *Occasionally in sexual abuse cases involving children, the aggressor is someone familiar to the child.*

In *most* sexual abuse cases, the aggressor is a relative, neighbor, or caretaker known to the child. Sexual abuse, rape, and incest are crimes. Children can and must be made to understand that while they need not be in a state of perpetual fear, they must be alert to unseemly sexual advances by any adult of either sex. Disabled children are particularly vulnerable targets for disturbed people. Children must be taught how to reject sexual advances as firmly and quickly as possible. Should a parent suspect that a child has been molested, or if a child tells a parent of sexual abuse, the parent has two crucial responsibilities. The first is to quietly and gently find out as much as possible about the incident. Children who, under pressure, felt caught in the moment and made to promise never to reveal a word must be told that promises made under such forced circumstances need not be kept. Having learned the details, parents must then in no way imply that the child was at fault. Sexual abuse is always the fault of the person who is older or more powerful than the child. Such careless remarks as "Why did you let him do this to you?" can be devastating. Children must be assured over and over again that nobody blames them for what happened. It has been found that many adults who suffer acute psychological distress as a result of having been molested during childhood are less disturbed by memories of the incident itself than by the possibility that they were somehow responsible for provoking it.

MYTH 45: *Young people who have thoughts about homosexuality are more likely to become homosexual adults.*

In spite of advances in psychology and medical research, we still do not know why any one person, male or female, is homosexual. There is certainly no evidence that girls who are tomboys and boys who prefer books to football are more likely to become homosexual adults. No longer is it thought that a child with a strong mother and weak father has a greater chance of becoming homosexual. What we suspect is that between four and ten percent of the population will have an exclusive homosexual orientation, no matter what parents try to do about it. Research indicates that an exclusive homosexual orientation is never a choice. It may be something that develops very early in a child's life, perhaps even before the age of two years, certainly before eight years. Some think it may be an inherited trait. A few have proposed that it is caused by a hormone imbalance before birth. Others think that a child's home environment, the way parents relate to one another and to their children, is the cause. No one really knows the answer. We don't even know if the homosexual orientation is permanent or if it's a condition that might be changed. Neither thoughts, nor fantasies, nor dreams, nor isolated homosexual experiences make one a homosexual. We do know that it's not contagious. One does not become a homosexual by knowing or being with someone who is.

In dealing with homosexuality, the messages that parents should convey are attitudes of consideration and understanding for people who have different orientations. Young people and adults can be very cruel with their language by implying homosexuality against a person they dislike. Besides the hurt it causes, it breeds a nasty and unwarranted prejudice that is carried over into adulthood. At the same time, parents should make it clear that their children are to reject any sexual overtures made by adults who most usually are pedophilic heterosexuals. Moreover, they must emphasize that such overtures do not suggest in any way that the child was somehow to blame. A child should be discouraged from thinking that he must be a homosexual simply because he was approached by someone who might be. It's a known fact that molestations and rapes are almost always by heterosexuals, rarely by homosexuals.

In the early Church, the Christian community was very rough on homosexuals because they thought they were freely choosing to go against nature. Today, the Church's attitude is changing. It teaches that the ideal form of sexual expression is between a man and a woman who are committed to one another for life and who are open to bringing children into the world. The Church also realizes that some persons are not to blame for circumstances that make them unable to attain the ideal. The Church does not approve of homosexual acts, but reserves judgment to God. The experience of homosexuals who remain in touch with the Church is helping Christians to be more understanding about their orientation.

Society's attitudes about homosexuality can seriously affect the development of young people. As parents, we need to convey messages that speak out against past prejudices and bigoted attitudes. It's wrong to make life difficult for people simply because they are different from us. It's just a fact that homosexuals can be happy and creative people, just as heterosexuals can turn to drugs and crime and lead unhappy lives. Since we believe that all of us were created in the image of God as "male" and "female," this emphasis requires our acceptance of male and female characteristics in each and every person. It also requires rejection of those stereotypes that degrade humanity and limit the potential of any man or woman, regardless of sexual orientation. When parents learn that their child is homosexual, they should remember that their child is still the *same* child they have always loved. They are the ones who have changed, by learning this fact new to them about their child. Never will their child need and deserve their love, understanding, and support more than from that moment on.

As Catholic parents, whether our children are gay or straight, we are challenged to witness to the Gospel message and imitate the Lord in all situations with charity and compassion.

MYTH 46: *Acquaintance rape occurs when the teenage girl does something to stimulate the boy.*

Rape is simply sexual intercourse forced on someone who does not wish it. It is a violent crime, and all violence is opposed not only to our Gospel values, but to all other human values. Rape is generally accompanied by threats or physical violence, and sometimes death. Although the act of rape involves the sex organs, it's an act of anger or aggression by a stronger against a weaker person. Until recently, women were made to feel that rape was somehow their fault, that they invited it by the way they dressed, walked, or acted. This is not true, and young women need to be informed to report such crimes. Rapists are being brought to trial more and more frequently as their victims gain the courage and support to testify. Most cities have sexual assault counseling services. If a woman is raped, she should call for advice about how to report the assault to the police as well as about getting help for her own natural feelings of fear and rage. We must never accept this kind of aggressive, dominant behavior from our male community. As parents, we are naturally afraid to think of this crisis ever happening to our daughters or our sons, remembering that almost all rapes are committed by heterosexual males. A clear message should always be sent that we are prepared to help. We don't want our children to suffer the additional hurt of being ashamed to seek help and support from those who love them most.

MYTH 47: *Chastity is a virtue which simply means that a person does not enter into physical, genital expressions of his or her sexuality.*

The virtue of chastity has a much broader and positive meaning than simply not participating in genital sexual activity. According to the Church teaching in the *Declaration on Sexual Ethics*, it is much more than that. "It is aimed at attaining higher and more positive goals. It is a virtue which concerns the whole personality, as regards both interior and exterior behavior." Chastity has both an interior and an exterior dimension. In its exterior dimension, what counts as chaste behavior depends on a person's lifestyle. For example, a particular form of behavior is expected from consecrated celibates, yet another form is proper for married persons, and still another for those living as singles. The directives for behavior imply that sexual-genital relations find their proper place only in marriage. In its internal dimension, chastity means the pure heart that does not lust. The best way to understand the virtue of chastity is that it enables the person to overcome the temptation to exploit other people sexually. More positively, we can say to young people that chastity enables a person to love unselfishly and have respect for others. Chastity is more than a law which prohibits sexual-genital relations between unmarried persons. It is our challenge to respond in a responsible and dignified manner in our relationships with persons of both genders.

MYTH 48: *Part of the problem of child pornography is that youngsters are willing to participate in such activities for the money.*

This is not true. "This sickness exists," says Father Bruce Ritter, founder of the New York City Covenant House, a non-profit youth shelter, "because a small segment of society wants it, another segment profits by it, and the rest aren't doing anything about it. Maybe we don't know enough—or care enough."

Each year as many as one million youngsters, ranging from the late teens to under a year, are sexually molested and then filmed or photographed either for the abuser's pleasure or for profit. Child pornographers are commercial operators who profit from the sickness of disturbed, immature people called pedophiles, who can receive sexual satisfaction only with children. Child pornographers often pick up youngsters who have run away from home. Their favorite subject is the attractive, smiling child—the more innocent looking, the better. Or pedophiles themselves may kidnap and molest a child, and then take photographs. Other children may actually be exploited by their own parents. Children may be lured into this by someone who is familiar, someone they are supposed to respect such as youth leaders, camp counselors, baby-sitters, or others in authority. The best way to protect your child is to give him or her clear warnings that no one, not even people in authority, should touch him or her in intimate ways. Insist that camps and organizations check the backgrounds on anyone who will be working with your child. Learn to recognize the signs of an assaulted child, which include chronic, unexplained physical complaints, loss of appetite, disturbed sleep, mood change, and sudden sexually-focused behavior. Never doubt if your child says that he or she has been molested; children are the victims of pornography and seldom lie about molestation.

Questions for Discussion

1. Have you ever been frightened by a sexual myth? What was it? Are there any dangers in holding on to it?
2. Is there anything in these myths you find difficult to accept?
3. Are there any people or institutions perpetuating some of these untruths?
4. What is our role as parents concerning these issues?
5. In what ways can you reflect God's true purpose of sexuality in your own family life?
6. Why are young people in need of guidance in their lives?
7. What is your impression of the way most parents encourage their children toward healthy, positive sexual lives?
8. What do you think you have to do to dispel some of these myths?
9. Does fear, embarrassment, or shyness ever keep you from seeking the truth?
10. How can we help ourselves and others like us who are sometimes afraid of their sexuality?

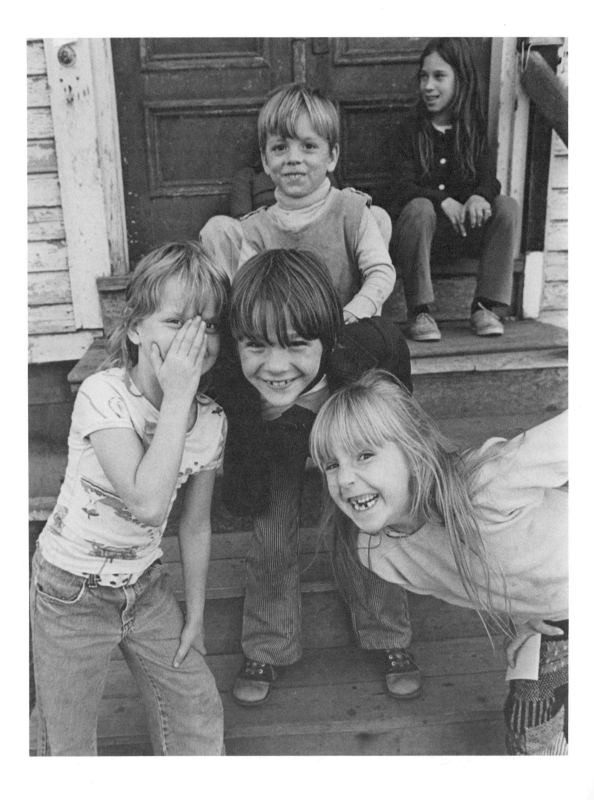

Child Development

As persons, each of us is unique. Our exact heredity, experiences, and potentials can never be duplicated. Even the closest of twins know that they have separate identities. But there are many things we do have in common. The structure and growth of our bodies all follow the same general patterns. The development of our minds and emotions, though subject to infinite small variations, follows predictable patterns. These patterns of growth and development are especially regular and pronounced in our earlier years. Knowing what to expect in these stages can help parents understand their children better. They can then be ready to supply what their children need at appropriate times.

Parents often suffer anxiety, confusion, and sometimes guilt about a particular turn their child's behavior has taken. A teacher, as an outside observer, can see that this happens most often at the transitions. As children take each step out of a comfortable and familiar childish stage into a more challenging and mature stage, parents grow gray hairs. With a little information and forethought, these transitions can be recognized and planned for, to become smoother and less stressful on the whole family. Parents can help each of their young ones meet the challenges of Christian life by preparing them with self-esteem, affirmation, values and facts.

Education in sexuality, as with most aspects of Christian life, is more caught than taught. Children learn by seeing, hearing, and absorbing what goes on around them, not just what is directed at them. They learn much by feeling the moods within the home. Their ways of understanding and thinking are not the same as those of adults. Their lack of knowledge, experience, and skill can cause great tension. They have little control over anything. For a very young child, almost every new experience can be frightening. For a teenager, love takes on new and often terrifying aspects. For those who have passed these stages, the experience may now be the first job interview, divorce, widowhood, or old age. For adults, these traumatic events are usually well-spaced, with recovery time in between. For young children, change may be constant. Until about sixteen to eighteen years of age, a large number of these changes originate within the body and are inescapable.

Young children have little ability to evaluate the things that happen to them or around them. They simply and uncritically absorb everything as fact. It is not until very late childhood that they can even begin to make critical judgments, feeling stronger and more secure in accepting some impressions and rejecting others. Children assemble ideas in ways that adults may think illogical. They are trying to cope with incomplete information and immature understandings. The results are sometimes humorous and sometimes sad.

Earlier we told of a fifth grade girl who believed she was pregnant. She was experiencing an important stage of clarifying and synthesizing facts about herself she had been collecting for years. Fortunately her mother did not poke fun at her, but was able to help her with this process to live through a minor crisis.

It would be more interesting to turn this story around and think of the mother as the main character. She was shocked when the whole situation came out in the open. It was difficult at first, but she was eventually able to sort out her daughter's misinformation and faulty reasoning. One cannot help but wonder how the story would have developed if this mother were prepared in advance. Suppose she knew the things that would have been on her child's mind at that age, and had prepared herself with knowledge, ready to guide her daughter toward new understandings. Wouldn't it have been nicer if she could have talked to her daughter earlier, without that twinge of horror in the back of her mind saying, "What has she done? Who has told her about getting pregnant? What does she know about intercourse?"

In the realm of sexual knowledge, children are learning from the moment of birth. As they learn to talk, some may ask lots of questions. Others, because they are naturally shy or for other reasons, may not ask. Wise parents will prompt children's questions when the time is appropriate—which is always earlier than most parents want. They will be aware of the opportunities for active growth in both knowledge and attitudes, and take advantage of them.

Volumes have been written about the ways children grow. From Sigmund Freud through Dr. Spock, Piaget, Kohlberg, Erikson, and many others, we have gained invaluable insights into the early years of life. This stock of knowledge is still growing. No one work could attempt to give a realistic synthesis of all of these researchers' findings. The following material is simply an overview of the high points as they relate to the sexual growth of children into young people. We hope that many of you will someday explore this topic in greater depth. It is an exciting and rewarding field of knowledge.

Age 0–1¹/₂ Years

Imagine having to get to know intimately several new people who have tremendously greater power than yourself, but on whom you depend completely. Imagine learning a new language, living in a new environment with lights and sounds and smells that you have never experienced. Imagine having no memories, no names for the objects around you, no idea what the parts of your body are or how they work. You probably can't recall the experience, but you were once in just this situation. All infants come into the world like this. They have to adjust to and learn virtually everything. They depend totally on their parents or parent substitutes to fulfill their needs.

Growing to well-rounded sexual maturity (sexualization) begins shortly after conception. Most body systems begin to function in the normal way that they will serve the person throughout life. Thought patterns begin to develop as baby begins to sense and cope with his or her environment. The physical and mental aspects of sexuality also begin their long development toward adulthood.

Shortly after birth, a boy baby experiences the erections he has been having regularly since the fourth month. Similarly, girls secrete lubrication within their vagina. These events are perfectly normal and they are the signs of normal, healthy sexual response. Both of these events will continue throughout the new person's life, if other factors don't inhibit them. This information often surprises parents. A boy's erection is quite visible but may be embarrassingly attributed to the "cold air" during a diaper change. The thought of a genuine sexual feeling in an infant horrifies many parents. That we are created sexual from conception is an idea many will agree to in print, but experience quite differently. The similarly early sexual functioning of girls is even harder for some adults to deal with, but the myth of the "unsexual" pre-adolescent girl cannot be sustained.

Babies must have all of their needs met by other persons. They tend to be quite self-oriented. But in infancy and early childhood this is healthy and normal. They are sense-oriented and won't be able to think in abstract terms until about age sixteen. The fulfillment of sensory needs must therefore be a prime concern for parents of infants. Studies have shown how infants, deprived of touching, hugging, soothing sounds, and interesting objects to look at, do not grow as rapidly or as satisfactorily as those with generous amounts of human caring and stimulation. Do we not, even as adults, crave the touch of others—the handshake of friends, the "hello" embrace of relatives, the caress of a spouse?

Mothers and fathers often delight in holding their newborn infants against their skin, caressing them, feeling every tiny finger and toe, the soft downy hair, and smooth little bottom. To mother this may seem a luxury; to baby it is essential. This is the beginning of the bond of love and trust between parent and child. This is the beginning of baby's feelings of acceptance and self-worth. These elements of acceptance and self-esteem are needed in all areas of development, including sexualization. As baby's vital needs for warmth, food, dry diapers, and cuddling are met, he or she grows in ability to trust and later on to become trustworthy.

A frequent snag in the acceptance and growing self-worth process comes when baby begins to explore his or her body. Fingers and toes, even mouth and nose seldom seem to be a problem, but woe to the infant who discovers a penis or vagina at bath time. Parents' own fears and apprehensions about the goodness of God's creation are operating when they push or slap the child's hand away or get the new diaper on as quickly as possible. Subtle messages of "You are dirty ; we don't like that part of you" are passed to baby. Self-esteem is hindered. Self-knowledge is hindered. Normal sexualization and later sexual functioning are put in jeopardy. No infant has the capacity to sin, but is only following the normal processes of discovery and growth created by God in all human beings.

Another part of the sexualization process is developing a gender identity. "It's a boy" or "It's a girl" signals the start of this development. Mom and dad usually respond with joy no matter what the sex of their child. But from the moment of that glorious announcement, some almost inevitable attitudes begin to take shape. How many young mothers are dismayed when they receive six pink baby blankets and then have a boy? Or how often does someone stop a young couple in the supermarket and remark of a young son, "What lovely, curly hair on your little girl!" Occasions like this make us chuckle inwardly precisely because we have ingrained in ourselves what we feel appropriate for a boy or girl. From the moment of birth, mom and dad and family and world will put expectations on the little one. Many of these are good and necessary. It is important for a child to grow into understanding what it means to be a male or female, for problems, from mild to severe, result from *not* understanding the proper sexual functioning of an adult man or woman. But equally serious problems can result from the extreme narrowing of the occupational, emotional, political, academic, spiritual, and other roles of males and females. Fathers often respond differently to a boy or girl baby. Girls receive more cuddling and gentleness; boys receive more verbal interaction and less caressing. A mother's feelings about her own sexual functioning or about her spouse's may subtly influence the way she treats her girl or boy infant. A mother may give confusing messages to her infant son if she resents her husband's sexuality for making her pregnant. She may feel that the sexuality of a daughter is a burden and a shame to be denied and avoided as long as possible.

Infants are great "receivers." Parents are laying the foundation for the child's whole life in these first two years. Many things are subtly begun now that will only come into flowering much later.

1¹/₂–3 Years

Children from about one and half to three years old are active explorers and "doers." From the earliest development of language through the "terrible twos," they keep their parents jumping. This is the age of becoming independent in the sense of being a separate self from the "others" and "things" around them. The word "no" screamed at high volume lets mom and dad know that the goal now is autonomy, at least to some degree.

Muscle control continues to develop and toilet training can begin at around two, but usually isn't reliable until three years of age and often later. It's important that parents realize the length of time this often takes and how much their child needs to feel that he or she is succeeding in this task. If expectations are too high or reprimands too severe, the youngster will certainly not feel autonomous, self-esteem will suffer and emotional growth will not progress at a healthy speed. But wait! What does toilet training have to do with sexuality? Remember, sexuality cannot be separated out from the rest of our lives and activities. That little boys can be a success at urinating when and where mom wants them to naturally leads to urination standing up, "like men do." Here is a small piece in the puzzle of gender identity. Toilet training, begun too early and too demandingly, can become a family crisis leading to negative feelings about the genitals, and about the need and ability to cooperate with the rest of the family. This leaves a child with feeelings of shame and self-doubt that are very hard to overcome.

As children learn to control muscles, to crawl, walk, talk, and evoke consistent reactions from family members, they also explore controlling their physical feelings. At a very young age most children masturbate, which often causes anxiety and embarrassment for parents. Parents bring to this situation their own histories of sexual learning and experience. Children only know they have discovered something about themselves that feels good, and they don't depend on someone else for it. They have control. But what is a parent to do? This often happens in the supermarket, or, even worse, when grandma comes to visit. It is important for us, as Christians, to control the flood of fears we have about masturbation and think, "Can a child this age really commit a sin?" Most definitely not. Masturbation and the accompanying sexual feelings are a normal part of growing up. Children who experience constant reprimand for touching their bodies at this age will most likely develop problems with later sexual functioning.

Children's understanding of their own and others' sexuality at this age is entirely simplistic and innocent. They will know for sure that they are a boy or a girl, but they may not be able to give a good reason why. Unless parents have instructed them or they have had a chance to ask about different bodies, they will give answers like "I'm a boy because I have short hair" or "I'm a girl because I like to play with dolls." This is the time to learn, very clearly, that all boys have a penis for urinating and later for passing sperm from the body. This is the time to learn that girls never have penises but do have a vulva, a vagina, and a uterus so that as grown women they might carry a baby. Children should have a chance to see the body of a child of the other sex, especially at moments when questions can be carefully guided and answered by a parent. Baby brother's or sister's bath time is perfect. Perhaps a visit to the home of a friend who has an infant can be arranged. If the child has these opportunities to learn but does not ask, it is important that parents give the information in a casual, matter-of-fact way. A child's firm understanding of the difference in external genitals at this age will eliminate much confusion and the possible later fear that a boy may lose his penis in some way, or that girls are inferior because they are missing something that other people have.

Understanding the process of reproduction beginning between age two and three hinges on the mental development of the child. At first, children cannot really grasp "past" or "future" ideas. Everything is here and now. They don't yet understand the concepts of growth or cause and effect. They cannot imagine a time before they were born. If you ask a child of two where babies are before they come into families, well, they must be at the hospital. What about before they were in the hospital? Baby heaven. This is natural and normal thinking. As their thought processes slowly develop, children will collect facts and tidbits of information and misinformation, often from older children. They will put these together in the best way they can. This often results in stories, concepts and statements that are hilarious to adults. But the children are dead serious; that is how they have figured it all out and believe it is. Parents should not laugh at these concepts nor push to move their child through this development too fast. Nor should they give up on giving correct information on the grounds that "the kid won't understand anyway." Very simple, correct information repeated often and lots of patience are the needs for this age.

Age 3–5 Years

Children of three to five are becoming rapidly more conscious of the world around them. Their curiosity and heightened sense of awareness now lead to almost constant questions. Many of these will naturally concern some aspect of sexuality. Also, few of these questions are whispered. They are most often delivered at full volume, and usually in the presence of strangers while shopping, or when the boss and his wife have come to dinner. How to deal with these uncomfortable situations is taken up in more detail in the section on talking about sex, but the basic rule is that the answers when given should be totally truthful, using correct names and terms.

Most questions at this age are fairly general and center on anatomical differences, pregnancy and birth. About this time, children have reached the "manufacturing" level of understanding reproduction. They realize that babies have not always existed but must be made. They think of them as having to be built rather than as growing. They have a very weak idea of the father's role in reproduction and often fall into the digestive fallacy: "It was something mommy ate that made the baby in her tummy," or "My mommy is making a baby. Whenever she eats the baby gets bigger." Though not always, this can sometimes lead to problems and fears later as children approach puberty. Remember the fifth-grader who thought she was pregnant? How did she think she got pregnant? We'll leave you to imagine. More commonly, young girls will confuse reproductive functions with those of the bowels. After all, both are located in a single, relatively small area of the body. This can lead to associating a sense of dirtiness and disgust at the normal menstrual process, a sense of reluctance toward being a woman and a generally lower self-esteem. Parents should give a clear message that nothing about the human body is dirty, bad or shameful—only private.

Children from about three to five years old are in the final stages of setting the foundation of their gender identity. They will explore many adult roles in what is called "rehearsal play." These often take the form of playing "house" with someone being the mother, the father, the child, and other characters. Parents often become upset when, during this rehearsal play, they find their son, Tommy, with an apron on, trying out the role of mother. This is normal. Tommy is firming up in his mind what a mother's role is. By experiencing this play, he is also clarifying for himself that the mother's role is not really for him, though fathers can do some things mothers can and vice versa. In the same day, he may also play at being a father, a fireman, a nurse, a doctor, a child, and maybe even the family dog. This experience is essential to healthy emotional growth and should not be prevented. Girls have always been allowed to play with dolls to practice their adult roles. Happily, now, toy manufacturers are making available a wide variety of small figures, more than just toy soldiers and glamor dolls, for both boys and girls to exercise their imaginations.

Another form of play common to this age group will certainly finish off any parents who have kept their cool so far. Most children, by age five, have still not satisfied their curiosity about their bodies, and will naturally seek to fill gaps in their knowledge. A wise parent or babysitter will deal very gently with children playing "doctor." This kind of play should probably not be allowed to continue at random, primarily because of the reactions of other parents. Neither should the children be scolded or made to feel that they have done something wrong. They can be gently distracted with cookies and milk, a TV show, or another game without instilling any of the guilt that can grow to debilitating proportions later in life. Avoiding this basic guilt and developing the sense of initiative is the central emotional task of the three to five year old.

Parents often ask about the significance of the Freudian "Oedipus Complex" at this age. According to his theory, children are said to fall in love with, and wish to marry, the parent of the opposite sex. This may or may not be accompanied by some hostility and competition with the same sex parent. Modern specialists in child studies tend not to place so much importance on this theory as was once popular. But undoubtedly the child is finalizing his or her concept of self as male or female and exercising this knowledge in the acceptance of the marriage roles. Susie learns of married love first by observing her parents. She begins to know what to expect of a future husband from dad. Her dad is the first man to love her and accept her femininity. Parents must deal with this stage in a firm but gentle manner. It is unfair and incorrect to encourage the child who wants to get rid of dad and marry mom, even if the parents only do it in an amusing way. The child needs to be told that mom and dad are already married to each other, that they love each other very much and intend to stay married to each other. But mom and dad also love their children. Parents should also reassure their children that they will grow up to have spouses of their own some day. They need to model a Christian marriage with consistent loving roles for male and female. In this way, children will grow up confident of the goodness of marriage and of their future competence as a husband or wife. This sets the stage for both faithful Christian marriages and healthy sexual functioning.

Emotions become a significant factor at this age as children begin to identify and express them. The sometimes overwhelming tensions of childhood can now be distinguished and dealt with in constructive ways, with a little parental help. Fear of the monster under the bed, genuine envy of another child's toys, and anger at an unpopular decision all need to find acceptable outlets. Though children still have difficulty controlling themselves at this age, they can understand the difference between feelings and actions. They can say, "I hit baby sister because I was mad at her for taking my teddy bear." If parents guide their children in identifying the emotions behind their actions, they begin a solid foundation for later emotional health, self-control, and responsible decision-making. The three year old's monster under the bed may become a bleeding ulcer for the thirty year old who still can't identify the monster and put it to rest.

Age 6–9 Years

The world begins to take on a rational and logical order for the six to nine year old. Developing the ability to recognize cause and effect and how they differ should become evident through these years. In this stage of "industry" children tend to become avid and unquenchable learners with steadily increasing ability to assimilate and relate facts. When they first enter the school environment, they move into a much wider realm of opportunity. For the school setting will slowly draw the child's horizons out of the family into the wider world. New friends, new adults, new places, new experiences all enrich and challenge the child. Also, additional sources of sexual information and misinformation are opened up to the child as association with older children generally increases. Parents who take an active and supporting role in developing Christian attitudes can help their children develop feelings of competence. Questions may now come at an increased pace if the child feels comfortable in asking. The child may easily turn to other sources of information if parents have not yet formed a foundation for being "askable." If Tommy meets with shock and disgust when he repeats at home something that was written on the bathroom wall at school, he learns that it is more fun as well as more informative to ask the other boys about it.

A child's understanding of the reproductive process now sticks to ideas that are technically possible. Conception is like planting a seed, and they can now understand that a baby grows. They think that all living things, babies included, have wills and act purposefully on their own. A baby grows because it wants to, not because of a natural process. As a wider range of questions is asked, parents will need to answer in even greater detail. A child of nine, at the upper end of this age range, may need a clear-cut description of sexual intercourse: "A father puts the sperm inside the mother." "But how?" (Take courage!) "The father's penis gets firm and is stiff enough to fit into a special place inside the mother called a vagina. That's how God arranged it so the sperm could get in." "Does it hurt?" (Don't faint, parents! The worst is already over.) "No, it doesn't hurt. It feels happy and good. God made it one of the ways that mommies and daddies can show how much they love each other."

Responsibility around the home increases during this age. Parents will be wise to avoid distinguishing between jobs for boys and jobs for girls. Basic gender *identity* was set by age two, and thereafter children continue to refine their understanding of gender roles as males or females. Sexual discrimination can begin at a very early age. Parents are usually unaware when they might be reinforcing what are known as role stereotypes. In schools, girls in the upper grades are often deeply offended when they are left out of such chores as carrying boxes, setting up chairs, or sweeping up after an assembly. In fact, girls in the fifth, sixth and seventh grades are, for the most part, larger and stronger than boys of the same age and so better able to perform these tasks. Boys as well as girls need to have their occupational and social roles left open as they grow. How many of us had the endowment for and would like to have become a lawyer, a chef, a carpenter, a baseball player, a surgeon, or an artist if only our family had thought it acceptable for a boy or girl?

It is often at around six that the question of nudity and modesty comes up. Whatever the family tradition has been, it is best not to make sudden changes. Sometime during this three year age range, children develop their own natural sense of modesty. They want to take baths alone, to have the bathroom door closed when using the toilet, and to have privacy when changing clothes. Perhaps this is a result of a deeper understanding of society's attitudes toward the body or a new awareness of the self as sexual. Whatever the cause, the desire for privacy should be respected by the rest of the family. As children spend more time at their friends' homes, parents must be keenly aware that other families often have different customs regarding nudity and modesty. In one family a trip from the shower to the bedroom with no clothes on may be normal. In another family this may be considered immodest. Parents and older family members must be careful not to scandalize or put undue pressure on guests, remembering that the amount of clothes one wears is more a matter of family custom than of genuine morality. Parents should also teach their children to respect the beliefs and family rules when they visit other people's homes.

With a child's entrance into school and a much wider peer group, sexual slang will surely need to be dealt with. It is important in this situation to make clear to the child exactly what he or she is being asked not to do. Being disrespectful about sexuality does not make sexuality a bad thing. The child who innocently says "fuck you" at the dinner table needs to receive a calm explanation of what polite and impolite conversation is. For a six year old, this is about enough. A nine year old can grasp the ideas of being disrespectful about a good thing and using words that are putdowns for other people. Children have a natural tendency to make jokes of new and unusual words. They are also very sensitive to anger and shame expressed by others, no matter how subtly. In dealing with sexual language with children, a great deal of patience and acceptance of childish thought is needed.

Fantasies and daydreams are a part of the normal growth through this age. As a means of exploring future roles, escaping tension, or processing new information, fantasy in most forms is usually healthy and growth-promoting at this time. Only if the child begins to slip in school work or refuse normal family and social interaction should parents seek counsel about bringing the child's fantasy life back into balance.

A strong ambivalence toward the opposite sex and close identification with same sex peers and parents is characteristic of this age. This led Freud to his concept of "latency" which is often used to support the idea that children at this age have no interest whatsoever in their developing sexuality. This is no longer believed to be true by the majority of child psychologists. The "latency" idea has also been used as an excuse not to teach about sexuality at this time, just when children are most eager and open to learning of all kinds. Children at this age handle sexual facts with an ease and matter-of-factness that can diminish as puberty approaches, so the years five to ten are best for providing full information on sexual matters, *before* puberty takes over.

Children are now learning to make promises. They begin to understand them as statements of fidelity to one's word and to the person to whom the promise was made. When a promise is broken, a child can be helped to deal with the failure by making amends for it. In this way, the groundwork for permanence in marriage and loving relationships is begun. Children also begin to rehearse social skills absorbed in the past. They can show "give and take" in peer friendships and dealings with adults. They slowly begin to realize social and emotional implications of sexuality, though their understandings are still very different from those of a teen or an adult. They are very sensitive to media influence and begin to be more aware of the sexual messages that the media impart. Conversations between parents and children of all ages about any confusing matter will make for solid mutual trust before puberty.

As the end of this age approaches, parents need to be preparing their children for the changes of puberty, because some girls begin menstruating at nine years old. For a girl to experience her first menstruation without adequate preparation is terrifying and a crime against love on the part of her parents. Increase in the growth of hair under the arms and in the pubic area, growth in breast size, and an increase in normal vaginal discharge are some of the signs of the imminence of the onset of menstruation. Boys of seven and up should be assured that it is normal to have frequent erections, and should also be prepared for the occurrences of wet dreams. All the normal physical changes of puberty need to be understood in advance of the occurrence. Parents who work to overcome their own admitted fears in order to prepare their children for puberty are appreciated by their children for carrying on an important task of parenthood and will earn the respect of their children for their efforts.

Age 10–12 or 13 Years

This is the age of dramatic hormonal changes. These hormones have been present in small amounts throughout the childhood years, but in the pre-teenager a rapid rise begins in their production. With this come the growth spurts, beginning first in girls and six months to a year later in boys. Awkwardness of body and emotion are to be expected. The most severe awkwardness is social because each individual's body timing is a little different from everyone else's. Pre-teens suddenly find that while they all looked like teddy bears before, now they all begin to look different. Some are getting bigger; some aren't. Some are getting rounder and some are getting pointier. Some are bony, some get their period or ejaculation, some just get acne, and mostly everyone gets confused. There is great concern with being normal, and so there is great comparison. Children are entering a critical time of testing their self-esteem. It's tough to know if you're okay when everyone is so different. You cannot be sure what okay really is.

Within the peer group, wide gaps may form between the girls and the boys. As girls are usually about one to two years ahead of boys in their physical development, they are also ahead of boys socially and emotionally. Girls will become interested in boys before the reverse happens. This often results in a time of "pressure" for the boys when the girls' expectations in games and friendships are quite different from their own. Boys may voice these concerns to their parents in subtle ways: "The girls are sure dumb lately . . . they're no fun to play with anymore." Girls sense this time lag in boys who, they feel, only want to do "rough" things and are self-centered and boring. Both boys and girls would benefit greatly by a simple explanation of what is happening to them at this time. They need to know that boys and girls are not worlds apart, but only a short time apart. They need to be helped not to develop negative attitudes toward the other sex, for these could remain to hinder their later social, emotional, and sexual growth. The "tomboy" girl or less-sports-minded boy may suffer especially at this age and need constant reassurance and guidance.

Children can now begin to think in both concrete and abstract ways. They can categorize and think ahead, and they can understand cause and effect and progressive development. They are collectors and fact gatherers, and will ask detailed, specific questions and expect truthful answers. Their peer group and the media have increasing influence now and provide more opportunities for information gathering and value formation. Though they may want to know all the details of pregnancy, birth and intercourse (in that order of importance), they do not yet understand the emotional involvement and implications which people just a few years older are well aware of.

During the pre-teens, friendships outside the home become ever more important. These friendships are often stormy as a new sense of identity, tolerance, and the old self-centeredness ebb and flow. This is the age of cliques at school. Girls discover the telephone and the latest styles. Boys immerse themselves in sports, teams, clubs, and hero worship. In striving for their independence, they yearn to become individuals but are not yet willing to give up the security of the family. This slow shift from family to peer group influence is a normal step toward adulthood and can cause relationships with other family members to begin to change. Daughters who were once close to their fathers now occasionally run to their room in tears leaving dad bewildered, wondering what he said. Boys become more private and may begin to keep more and more of their emotions to themselves, sharing less with the family.

As pre-teens begin to test the old rules and expectations of family life, their parents' anxiety level tends to rise. Children may now try their first cigarette, or sneak their first taste of beer or wine. Some give in to pressures to experiment with drugs. It is very difficult for parents to accept that children who look so young are really making their first hesitant moves out of the nest. Children change inwardly more than their external bodies show. Teachers at the later middle school and junior high grades often have to deal with parents who are frightened and confused or feel out of control, guilty or angry. Often they see these "rebellious" activities of their children as an indication of their own failure to raise them properly. How parents react at this stage is crucial. Now is the time to make special efforts to keep communication open and to boost children's self-esteem by trusting the children more and more with solid information about all personal matters. Good family values and ideals need to be reaffirmed. Children need to be reassured that their curiosities and friendships are normal. They need to know that they are still loved by the family, even as they try their wings and seek to withdraw from it. They need to know that their physical development, no matter how out of time with their peers' it may seem, is normal and healthy. The key note should always be, "We love you and believe in you. We may not always agree with you or approve of what you do, but our love for you cannot change, and we're always ready to talk with you about puzzling things."

Age 12–14 or 15

These ages are purposely overlapped because this shift from childhood into adolescence is just not clear-cut. The first menstruation or first wet dream is a milestone, to be sure, but does not of itself make a whole new person. As children become teens, the tendencies that began stirring in the pre-teen years begin to develop faster. Changes begin to happen more rapidly, especially in boys. Hormones may fluctuate widely. Bodies become more adult-like, but not all at once, and not evenly. Differences in body structure between individuals and variations within each individual can cause great concern. Whereas girls who grew and menstruated earlier may now begin to feel comfortable with themselves, some girls will not begin to menstruate until the end of this age. Some boys will begin to shoot up, grow out of three sizes of $30 jeans in a year and experiment with their father's razor. Other boys will still look like teddy bears at age fourteen. Occasionally, younger siblings may outgrow their older brothers or sisters during this time. This is a delicate family situation to handle, requiring awareness, sensitivity, and special caring from busy parents. By about fourteen or fifteen, most teen bodies are fully functional sexually. They are now biologically able to be parents—a profound responsibility added to their growing lives.

New emotions come to the surface at this age. As sexual feelings of arousal become evident and intense, guilt and anxiety may increase. Early teens begin to understand the emotional implications of intercourse on a primary level. They may have intense curiosity about this. Correct information about both the physical and emotional aspects of sexual intercourse can help satisfy curiosity, calm fears and often actually prevent early experimentation. When teens feel secure in knowing about something, they don't have to try it out in secret.

As teens separate themselves from parents to an ever greater extent, peer relationships become more and more important. Teens begin to practice adult roles and experiment with more mature attachments. As they begin dating, relationships have the potential to become longer and more intense. Same-sex friendships are still more numerous than dating friendships, however, and as these same-sex friendships can be very intense they often raise anxieties in parents about possible homosexual feelings and acts. It is common for persons at this age to develop an interest in the bodies of others of the same sex. This may be due to curiosity about sexuality in general and a concern about one's own development as part of the normal learning process of life. Parents may need to discuss this with their teens. This discussion should, of course, be calm and easy-going. The teens need to know that they are normal. They need to have their fears and misconceptions put to rest. This is not the time for parents to air their own hostilities or fears about adult homosexuality, which is another matter entirely. Less than ten percent of people have a homosexual orientation, and that will be dealt with elsewhere in this book. Parents need not add this complex problem to all the others that teens have during this age. They should be earnestly striving to lessen the stresses of growing up, not add to them.

Parents should not assume that young people have a clear grasp of everything involved in their own growth process. Continued information, guidance and support are essential. Christian values can be affirmed and seen from a more mature perspective as teens grow. Curiosity and questions begin to shift from biological interests to a concern with moral implications. As young teens test their childhood beliefs and values, they often find themselves in conflict situations, and great hurts are possible at this time. Exploitation and manipulation by the media are real threats. Teens need access to other trusted adults as well as their own parents to provide some sense of stability and to remind them of their uniqueness and goodness in the eyes of God.

All factual knowledge about the physical workings of our sexual selves should be available to early teens. Things that were earlier just mentioned will usually need to be more fully discussed now that they can be seen in a new light. Bodily changes need to be reviewed as they are about to happen, as they are beginning, and as they are in full force. Dad needs to be gentle with the boy who dulls his razor. Mom needs to be tenderly sensitive to the genuine importance of a girl's first real date, even if it is only a trip to the hamburger stand. Acne and awkwardness need gentle acceptance and concern. A sense of perseverance and patience should be conveyed to early teens. Size is a very common complaint of early teens—"I'm too tall" "I'm too short" "My breasts won't grow" "What's the matter with me? I can't get my pants zipped comfortably." Fussing and fretting is characteristic of the early teen.

Hygiene relating to sexuality is a major concern for teens who are experiencing this for the first time. Both girls and boys need plenty of warmth and support from their parents. All the little extras, like not leaving the sanitary supplies out on the bathroom shelf to protect a shy girl from a curious younger brother, or changing a boy's bedsheets without complaint or implied criticism, will be deeply appreciated. Acceptance of sexuality as natural and good can co-exist with respect for the often shy and unsure feelings of young teens.

Age 15–18

During the late teen years, parents' control and formation of their children is now shared with the larger community and is often effectively out of their hands. Parents need to understand, accept and interact with this. Older teens need freedom for risk-taking and decision-making. When sometimes the young person exhibits quite mature reactions, comment and approval are required. When at other times he or she reacts almost as a child, love and support are needed. All teens need to have their budding adult identity affirmed and supported, and this is when adult behaviors and privileges can be assumed to an increasing degree, so that a sense of personal responsibility can be developed. This should be based on the Christian values absorbed by children over the past fifteen years, adequate knowledge of their bodies, and a belief in their own goodness conveyed by parents and community.

The late teen may often seem rebellious and reckless, but he or she will ultimately act on values absorbed in the past. If parents were present and active, their values showing through clearly during the years up to now, then they should not be surprised by their late teen's values. If parents were barely present, giving no examples of values, but only rigid legalisms, or passed on confused and conflicting values, then teens will turn elsewhere to find value systems they can hold. This "elsewhere" is most frequently the media—TV, records, or their peer group.

As young people move through this stage, they become tremendously idealistic. They are keenly aware of hypocrisy and rules that don't work. They have little tolerance for the ambiguities of adult life. They tend to swing toward the extremes in any situation. Parents who understand this idealism can be of great help in guiding their teens in sexual values. Most teens will have experienced not necessarily intercourse, but some genital sexual activity well before their late teens. Parents who can appeal to their child's sense of idealism are on the right track toward developing mature, Christian sexual behaviors. Parents who rely on legalisms, threats and fear tactics to prevent early sexual experience only alienate their children, turn them over to their peer groups, and make early intercourse probable and teen pregnancy possible. Parents can no longer control, but they can continue to teach and model their own values and, by keeping communication open, act as information and loving care givers.

Late teens face many of the sexual problems that are also experienced by adults—unwanted pregnancy, venereal disease, prostitution, the realization that one is a homosexual, broken relationships, lack of self-esteem. These are not easy things for adults to deal with, and for teens they are crises that have genuine life or death consequences. Bearing in mind the high suicide rate in teenagers, when problems like the above come into a family, parents need to have two primary understandings. First, parents do not make teens' choices for them. Parents must not be so guilt-ridden about their children's problems that they cannot provide effective help, guidance and love. Parents are not always responsible for the actions of their older teens. Second, parents are not forever expected to "go it alone" with their family's problems. There are many Church and community related helping agencies set up precisely because parents are not trained or prepared to cope with all the possible calamities this world can throw at them and their children. Parents who use these helping agencies, in spite of pride or fear, are giving their best to their children in setting aside self for love of their family in a truly Christian way.

To avoid these pitfalls, teens need advance knowledge and the freedom to seek new knowledge from parents and other reliable sources. Parents who have been open and askable all along now have the opportunity to speak again about the kind of love one needs for a lasting relationship, how to know if you have this, and what to do with a broken heart. They will not think that hearing their eighteen year old say he is gay is an easy situation to deal with, but they will be able to cope without driving their son away forever. They will be consulted to support and console their unwed teen mother, rather than lose her to an abortion clinic and possibly then to a pimp in another city. More often, they will just be there to be asked, "How did you feel when . . ." or "Will anyone really love me?" or "Gee, dad, why did she get so upset when I kissed her?"

It's sad to say that parents who haven't before talked with their pre-teens and young teens, who haven't become askable and open about sex, now have only a small chance of "catching up." Young people who have reached their later teens without bonds of communication with their parents are less likely to turn to them in times of crisis. When crises do arise in families without established communication, professional counseling can go a long way in helping develop a new foundation—if the family members are willing to try.

As people end their teens and move into their early twenties, parents have only a little direct influence over their decisions and behavior. If the children have left the household, they are, for all purposes, free to act on their own values. They enter the world of adults, taking at least the consequences if not the responsibility for their own actions. Parents who have tried to encourage healthy growth in sexuality, who have modeled their values clearly and consistently and who have kept lines of communication open will probably remain close to their children. Their children will continue to ask questions, call for advice, and share their secrets with them.

Questions for Discussion

1. Give some examples of how education in sexuality is more caught than taught at home.
2. How does more knowledge in how children develop sexually help parents?
3. How do very young infants normally exhibit sexual response?
4. What should be the primary concerns of parents regarding the healthy sexual growth of their infants?
5. What is "gender *identity*"? How does it develop through the first two childhood years? What is "gender *role*"? How have our concepts of it changed?
6. How does toilet training affect the feelings of autonomy and the sexual attitudes of children?
7. Why do children masturbate? What is its significance in the development of the child?
8. Describe how children's understanding of reproduction changes as they mature.

9. What is the importance of "rehearsal play" in children? When might parents feel this is a problem?
10. How can parents cope with the child who competes with one parent for the affection of the other?
11. How are parents helping their children's later emotional health when they help young children identify and deal with their emotions?
12. What factors outside the home begin to influence children's sexual learning as they grow past five years old? How can parents insure that they remain the most influential factor?
13. Why is it important to be aware of how children learn adult role potential? How do parents narrow or widen this potential?
14. When should parents begin to prepare their children for the physical and emotional changes of puberty? How can parents help to reassure their children that they are normal?
15. What are some of the particular problems of the pre-teen and early teen years?
16. What can parents do to keep communication going with their children throughout all the growing years to maturity?

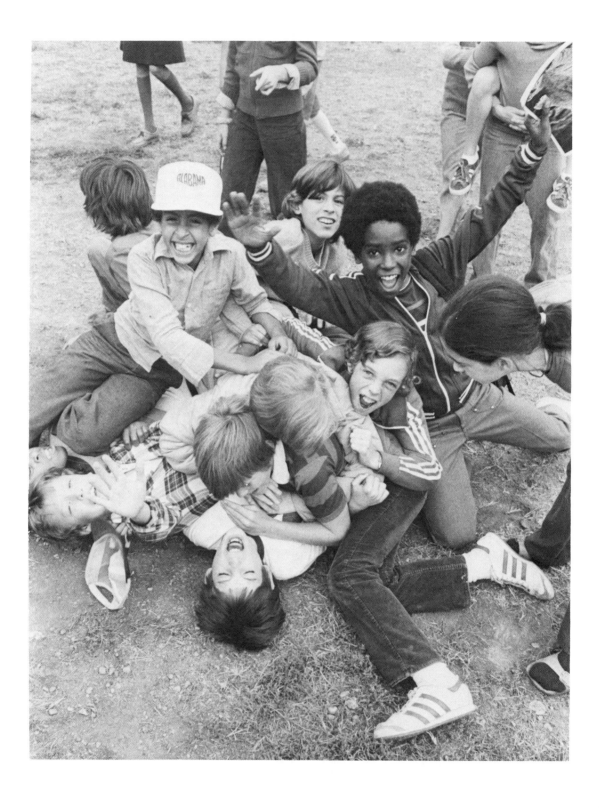

Sexual Knowledge

Parents don't need to be walking encyclopedias in order to live their lives successfully and teach their children as well, but answering questions with half-truths or myths can cause harm in later life, so a certain amount of accurate information about our bodies and how they work is certainly necessary. Knowledge of a little more than just the bare essentials can enhance any relationship, making people more secure, less open to exploitation, and more likely to be happy throughout their lives. Information can help people cope with crises that arise in their families as well as providing background for everyday decision making.

Parents Talk Love cannot begin to offer a comprehensive human biology course. It does not intend to. There are many excellent books that offer thorough information about the workings of our bodies and other current sexual questions. Every concerned adult or responsible parent should purchase one of these and have it handy in their home. Often we forget things we were once told and have to brush up on our understanding. New information, beyond what we were taught by our parents, is now available. Youngsters growing up usually need to have the same information presented several times before they can grasp the whole story and truly understand it. The chapter of resources will discuss the kinds of books available to fill various needs. Following is a basic outline of the kinds of information parents need to make available to their children as they grow up. For parents who never learned most of this material from a reliable source (don't feel bad—you're the norm, not the exception), it would be good to start in the earliest years and work your own way through this knowledge before presenting it to your children.

Just one caution: those of us who are over age twenty have had plenty of time to collect misinformation. The most caring and careful parents will throw away the idea, "I already know that," and check out each area of knowledge with a fresh openness to learning things they might have missed before.

The second half of this chapter presents a quiz-format, check-yourself exercise on some, but by no means all, currently relevant sexual information.

Following is an outline of the sexual knowledge needs of children at various ages:

The child 0–2 years old needs:

1. to know how it feels to be loved, touched, caressed, and held, and to trust in others (this is a very basic need which continues throughout all ages).

2. to observe love and physical affection, such as kissing and touching between his or her parents.

3. to hear the names of the genitals—penis, testicles, vagina, vulva and uterus—said along with all the other body parts.

4. to learn a basic sense of the goodness of his or her body, all its products, all its functions.

The child 2–5 years old needs:

1. to develop a sense of gender identity, to be sure that "I am a girl" or "I am a boy."

2. to know that all boys and men have penises and that this is never "lost" because of naughtiness or other behavior.

3. to know that all girls have vulvas and vaginas, never a penis or testicles, and that there is nothing "less" about a girl's sex organs as compared to a boy's.

4. to understand that all closed doors should be respected by everyone, children *and* parents.

5. to continue to observe parents' love and their respective roles in the home.

6. to observe other family members behaving in responsible ways.

7. to understand that babies come into families because of the love between parents.

8. to learn that all their body functions, elimination included, are normal and good.

9. to have a very basic idea of pregnancy and breast feeding.

The child age 5–8 years old needs:

1. to continue growing in gender role understanding and to explore various adult roles, e.g., mommy, daddy, nurse, doctor, fireman, musician, who's boss for this or that, whether daddies can cook and mommies can drive trucks?

2. to reconfirm the names and goodness of his or her sexual body parts—penis, testicles, scrotum, vagina, vulva, labia, breast, nipples.

3. to understand that a baby grows inside the mother, from a cell from the mother and a cell from the father.

4. to know that babies are born through their mother's vagina.

5. to continue to observe and assimilate signs of affection and trust, and to exhibit these toward parents and other family members.

6. to be given (both boys and girls) a basic understanding of menstruation. In the case of larger, more mature girls, this information is protective and particularly vital.

The child 9–11 years old needs:

1. a thorough introduction to female external and internal anatomy—labia, clitoris, hymen, vagina, uterus, fallopian tubes, ovary, ovum.

2. a thorough understanding of menstruation, the menstrual cycle, and menstrual hygiene.

3. an appreciation of the goodness of both male and female sexual functioning.

4. a thorough introduction to male external and internal anatomy—penis, scrotum, testes, glans, foreskin, circumcision, semen, vas deferens, seminal vesicle, cowpers and prostate glands.

5. a basic understanding of male and female sexual response, vaginal lubrication, male erection, ejaculation, and "wet dreams."

6. a deeper understanding of conception, pre-natal growth, and birth.

7. a knowledge of the changes that take place in adolescent bodies—growth of axillary hair, breast development, bone and muscle growth, voice change, changes in skin, awkwardness.

8. a beginning understanding of the expected emotional, social and spiritual changes of adolescence.

9. a deeper understanding of family roles and responsibilities, social expectations, the role of affection and love.

The child age 12–14 years needs:

1. a basic understanding of the intensity of sexual feelings, human sexual response mechanisms, and their direction toward intercourse.

2. to begin to develop an understanding of the meaning of dating.

3. to begin to develop responsible strategies for coping with the strong sexual drives of the teen years.

4. to understand the potential for exploitation by the media and peers, and to develop strategies to cope with this.

5. to realize the significance of venereal disease in the teen population, to know the facts, and where to turn for help for himself or herself or to advise friends.

6. to have a clear understanding of the facts and implications of contraception.

7. to understand the procedures and implications of abortion.

8. to have up-to-date factual knowledge concerning homosexuality, its prevalence in society, and the statistical incidence of irreversible homosexual orientation, and to understand that homosexuals are among the least dangerous and most gifted and productive people in society.

9. reassurance that his or her sexual development and maturation is normal and healthy, that close friendships with the same sex at this age are normal, as are crushes on teachers or other adults, and that these are not indications of homosexual tendencies or abnormal sexual development.

10. a new presentation of the family's values in more mature terms.

11. constant reassurance that his or her new curiosity, new feelings, need to explore, to become independent, to take risks, are all a part of growing up and should be exercised within healthy limits.

12. constant knowledge that the family will not abandon him or her, but will continue to offer support on ever-maturing levels.

13. to be reassured that no physical damage is involved in masturbation and that if this poses a religious problem there are understanding and knowledgeable clergy who can help teens deal with this.

The child age 15–18 years needs:

1. ready access to all the factual material covered in previous stages, as facts are often forgotten when they are not immediately relevant.

2. a more sophisticated understanding of sexual anatomy and functioning.

3. a deeper understanding of the human sexual response systems and how emotion and physical sensation interact with each other.

4. to concretize and act on strategies for dealing with sexual drives in dating relationships.

5. to be clear in their values founded on those of their family, religious beliefs, social customs.

6. to be aware of non-family support for teens, in the form of community groups or Church support systems.

7. a deeper understanding of the role of sexuality in all relationships and various adult roles.

The person over eighteen is considered nearly an adult sexually, though a wide range of maturity and knowledge levels may still exist. If the eighteen year old has absorbed all the knowledge suggested so far, then the tasks of adult learning lie ahead.

Adults need:

1. to be able to identify questions concerning sexuality and search out answers from appropriate sources.

2. to recognize sexual dysfunction and seek competent counseling when necessary.

3. to integrate their sexuality into their whole person and into relationships with others.

4. to fulfill the roles of spouse, friend, parent where appropriate.

5. to exhibit values through responsible sexual behavior.

6. to act knowledgeably and positively when involved in sexuality-related cultural and societal conflicts, e.g., gay rights, women's lib, concern for the disabled and elderly.

7. to remain open to new learning through formal and informal educational opportunities and through experience.

Sexual Knowledge Activity

The following is a list of questions about sexuality-related topics. This by no means covers all the information an adult should know, but hopefully will serve to stimulate you to find out more about yourself as a sexual person. Some of the answers are less obvious and less certain. Test yourself. Then look into those questions you were a little shaky on, do a little research and learning.

1. When a female child is born, she already has all the egg cells she will ever have. She may normally begin to experiment with masturbation before one year of age and this should never be punished.

T. F.

2 When a male child is born, he is capable of experiencing an erection of the penis and may normally begin to experiment with masturbation before one year of age, and this should never be punished.

T. F.

3. Hormonal changes at puberty can cause:
   a. acne or pimples
   b. changes in the voice of both sexes
   c. increased perspiration and a need for deodorant
   d. all of the above

3. _____

4. Adolescent girls usually menstruate for about a year before they begin to ovulate.

T. F.

5. Adolescent boys usually begin to experience erection and orgasm before they begin to produce sperm cells.

T. F.

6. The woman's _____ is a small organ on the outside of her body that is sensitive to sexual stimulation.
   a. cervix   b. vesicle
   c. vagina   d. clitoris

6. _____

75

7. The man's _____ keeps sperm at a constant temperature by stretching and contracting, thereby raising (to warm) and lowering (to cool) the testicles.
   a. vas deferens
   b. scrotum
   c. testes
   d. cowper's gland

   7. _____

8. About once a month, an egg is released from a woman's ovary in a process called:
   a. ejaculation
   b. ovulation
   c. fertilization
   d. menstruation

   8. _____

9. The release of sperm and seminal fluid through the penis is called:
   a. ejaculation
   b. ovulation
   c. fertilization
   d. menstruation

   9. _____

10. The lining of the uterus grows thick each month in preparation for a pregnancy. If no pregnancy occurs, the lining is shed in a process called:
    a. ejaculation
    b. ovulation
    c. fertilization
    d. menstruation

    10. _____

11. The meeting of sperm and egg is called:
    a. ejaculation
    b. ovulation
    c. fertilization
    d. menstruation

    11. _____

12. Women usually ovulate about two weeks before a menstrual period but some may also ovulate when stimulated by sexual intercourse.

    T. F.

13. Eggs are released from the ovary and are available for fertilization for about:
    a. 2–4 hours
    b. 12–24 hours
    c. 2–4 days
    d. 5–7 days

    13. _____

14. Sperm cells are deposited in the vagina during intercourse, and travel through the cervix into the uterus, where they remain viable for:
    a. 2–4 hours
    b. 12–24 hours
    c. 2–4 days
    d. 5–7 days

    14. _____

15. When an egg is fertilized in the fallopian tubes, it travels to the uterus and implants in the uterine lining. Implantation usually occurs about _____ after fertilization.
    a. 2–4 hours   b. 12–24 hours
    c. 2–4 days   d. 5–7 days

    15. _____

16. Early sexual encounters can jeopardize later development of good sexual relationship in marriage.

    T. F.

17. Alcohol and drugs can inhibit sexual response.

    T. F.

18. Effective stimulation of the clitoris is important in achieving orgasm in women.

    T. F.

19. A man's sexual performance is related to the size of his penis.

    T. F.

20. When a woman is sexually aroused, all of the following are normal reactions *EXCEPT:*
    a. nipples become erect   b. vagina is lubricated
    c. pulse rate increases   d. clitoris emits liquid

    20. _____

21. Erections of a man's penis can be caused by:
    a. visual stimulation
    b. touching and caressing
    c. thoughts and fantasies
    d. all of these

    21. _____

22. Simultaneous orgasm enhances fertility.

    T. F.

23. Which of the following causes sexually transmitted disease (STD)?
    a. injury   b. body strain
    c. bacteria or virus   d. poor hygiene

    23. _____

24. Syphilis and gonorrhea can be cured by using
    a. ultraviolet light   b. vitamin E
    c. bed rest   d. antibiotics

    24. _____

25. Many women and some men who have STD don't notice any symptoms.

T. F.

26. Syphilis can remain in a person's body for many years without symptoms, but it can be detected at any time by a:
    a. Pap test
    b. blood test
    c. pelvic exam
    d. saliva test

    26. _____

27. Untreated gonorrhea can cause sterility because of:
    a. infections in the bladder
    b. scar tissue in the vas deferens
       or fallopian tubes
    c. damage to the uterus but no damage in men
    d. changes in the levels of hormones
       produced by the gonads

    27. _____

28. The surest way to prevent infections from venereal disease is:
    a. kill all mosquitos
    b. avoid public toilets
    c. take daily showers
    d. avoid skin contact with infected persons

    28. _____

29. The venereal disease called "Herpes II" is:
    a. a virus, much like cold sores
    b. related to birth defects and
       possibly cervical cancer
    c. incurable at this time
    d. all of the above

    29. _____

30. Most birth control pills work by preventing the ovaries from releasing any:
    a. hormones
    b. eggs
    c. sperm
    d. menstrual fluid

    30. _____

31. In order to work properly, a woman must take a birth control pill:
    a. each time she has sex
    b. each time she has orgasm
    c. each time she ovulates
    d. every day for three weeks each month

    31. _____

32. A woman using an IUD may experience:
    a. headaches and breast tenderness
    b. increased menstrual cramps and flow
    c. more frequent need to urinate
    d. all of the above

32. _____

33. A couple who wish to use natural methods of family planning will probably be asked to:
    a. take the woman's temperature
       every morning for several months
    b. check the woman's cervical mucus
       daily for several months
    c. keep careful track of the woman's periods
       for several months
    d. all of the above

33. _____

34. Natural family planning (NFP) methods of birth control work when:
    a. the woman has irregular cycles
    b. the woman doesn't have intercourse
       during her fertile times
    c. sickness interrupts the cycle
    d. the woman is very young

34. _____

35. Withdrawal as a birth control method is:
    a. frustrating   b. better than nothing
    c. about 75% effective   d. all of the above

35. _____

36. Douching is not a good birth control method because:
    a. sperm are already in the uterus
    b. it is too expensive
    c. the vagina is too big
    d. sperm swim faster in cold water

36. _____

37. A/An _____ is placed inside a woman's uterus to prevent implantation of fertilized ovum.
    a. IUD   b. condom
    c. pill   d. diaphragm

37. _____

79

38. The _____ is placed inside a woman's vagina to prevent sperm from entering the uterus.
    a. IUD   b. condom
    c. pill   d. diaphragm

                                                    38. _____

39. Which of these may cause side effects because it works through the bloodstream?
    a. IUD   b. tubal ligation
    c. pill   d. condom

                                                    39. _____

40. Condoms are an effective method of birth control because:
    a. they get men involved in contraception
    b. they help prevent venereal disease
    c. they prevent sperm from entering
       the woman's body
    d. all of the above

                                                    40. _____

41. A woman can never get pregnant from having intercourse during her period.

                                                    T. F.

42. The success of a birth control method depends largely on the motivation of the couple using that method.

                                                    T. F.

43. Twins are caused by:
    a. two sperm fertilizing one egg
    b. one sperm meeting two embryos
    c. either two sperm and two eggs or one
       fertilized egg that split in two

                                                    43. _____

44. Natural childbirth means birth without:
    a. hospitals   b. doctors
    c. much medication   d. prenatal classes

                                                    44. _____

45. A pregnant woman can usually have sex safely:
    a. for the first three months only
    b. until two or three weeks before delivery
    c. only in the fourth and fifth months

                                                    45. _____

46. Most victims of sexual abuse are attacked on the street by strangers:

                                                    T. F.

47. Most children who are victims of non-violent forms of sexual misconduct will be harmed in their later development.

T. F.

48. Children are usually guilty of some form of seduction or encouragement in child sexual abuse cases:

T. F.

49. Women who are victims of rape always call the police or seek professional help.

T. F.

50. Police and community service personnel who deal with rape victims have the general attitude that it was the woman's fault for letting herself be raped:

T. F.

51. When an average boy goes through puberty:
    a. he loses his "baby fat" and becomes slimmer
    b. his penis becomes larger
    c. he produces sperm
    d. his voice becomes lower
    e. all of the above

51. _____

52. As part of the normal sexual functioning:
    a. two eggs each month are released,
       one from each ovary, in mature women
    b. millions of eggs each month are released
       from one ovary in mature women
    c. testes produce one sperm for each
       ejaculation (climax) in mature men
    d. none of the above

52. _____

53. It is true that:
    a. a large penis increases a woman's sexual enjoyment
    b. a large penis means a man is more sexually active
    c. a larger penis increases more in size
       when erect than a small penis
    d. women with small breasts do not enjoy sex very much
    e. size of body parts is not related to sexual enjoyment

53. _____

54. Masturbation (self stimulation):
    a. is something many males and many females do
    b. is something only males do
    c. is something only females do
    d. is something only a few males and
       a few females do
    e. none of the above

                                                        54. _____

55. If six year old boys look at each other's genitals while playing "doctor" or taking a bath:
    a. they will be bothered by the memory
       for the rest of their lives
    b. they will probably become homosexuals
    c. they will be pretty much the same
    d. they will be doing something not
       commonly done by young boys

                                                        55. _____

56. The sexual double standard means that:
    a. boys are rewarded for having sexual
    experiences while girls are punished for having them
    b. boys and girls are equally free to
       have sexual experiences
    c. boys and girls are equally punished
       for sexual experiences

                                                        56. _____

57. A person is a homosexual if that person:
    a. has a crush on a school teacher of the same sex
    b. enjoys hugging and kissing
       close friends of the same sex
    c. has very warm feelings for
       the parent of the same sex
    d. all of the above
    e. none of the above

                                                        57. _____

58. Temporary impotence among men may be due to:
    a. overuse of drugs and alcohol
    b. physical fatigue
    c. depression
    d. all of the above
    e. none of the above

                                                        58. _____

59. Young children usually play with each other sexually because:
    a. they are "turned-on" to each other
    b. they are naturally curious
    c. they have not been taught proper morals

    59. _____

60. Homosexuality is usually the result of:
    a. a passive father and a dominant mother
    b. a hormonal imbalance
    c. a genetic defect
    d. factors largely unknown

    60. _____

61. Teenagers sometimes avoid medical care for VD because:
    a. they do not recognize the symptoms
    b. they are afraid of the physical exam
    c. they have to report their sexual contacts
    d. all of the above

    61. _____

62. A man's role as the family provider and a woman's role as the homemaker are:
    a. totally determined by their biology
    b. mostly determined by biology but
        also influenced by society
    c. mostly determined by society but
        also influenced by biology
    d. totally determined by society

    62. _____

63. Treatment of venereal disease is best if:
    a. both partners are treated at the same time
    b. only the partner with the symptoms
        sees the doctor
    c. medication is taken only as long
        as the symptoms remain
    d. the partners continue their
        usual frequency of intercourse

    63. _____

64. As they enter puberty, teenagers become more interested in sexual activities because:
    a. their sex hormones are changing
    b. the media push sex for teenagers

c. some of their friends are having sex
and expect them to also
d. all of the above

64. _____

65. People who have sexual fantasies:
a. are usually unhappy with their sex life
b. act out most of their fantasies
c. have sex with many different partners
d. all of the above
e. none of the above

65. _____

66. Sexual fantasies are:
a. experienced by many men
b. experienced by many women
c. experienced by many adolescents
d. all of the above
e. none of the above

66. _____

67. Regarding the age of physical maturity:
a. girls usually mature several years earlier than boys
b. most boys mature several years earlier than most girls
c. all boys and girls are fully mature by age sixteen
d. all boys and girls are fully mature by age eighteen

67. _____

68. A woman *cannot* become pregnant:
a. the first time she has sexual intercourse
b. a few days after sexual intercourse
c. if she has sexual intercourse during her period
d. if she has sexual intercourse while standing up
e. if the male climaxes next to the opening
of the vagina, without having intercourse
f. none of the above

68. _____

69. When an average girl goes through puberty:
a. her breasts become developed
b. her hips become larger
c. she loses her "baby fat" and becomes slimmer
d. she grows body hair under her arms
e. all of the above

69. _____

70. Learning new information about human sexuality leads people to:
   a. become sexually promiscuous
   b. deny their sexuality
   c. think more fully about their sexuality
   d. none of the above

   70. _____

71. Physical feelings during intercourse are increased:
   a. by drinking a lot of alcohol
   b. by taking a lot of drugs
   c. by being free of guilt and nervousness
   d. none of the above

   71. _____

72. The boy most likely to boast about his sexual exploits is the one who:
   a. is very active sexually
   b. is worried about his masculinity
   c. is comfortable with his appearance
      and sexual activity

   72. _____

73. The physical changes of puberty:
   a. happen in a week or two
   b. happen to different children at different ages
   c. happen quickly for girls and slowly for boys
   d. happen quickly for boys and slowly for girls

   73. _____

74. Wet dreams are:
   a. a sign that a boy is thinking too much about sex
   b. shameful, and the boy should be encouraged
      to try not to have them
   c. a normal part of growing up and should be
      accepted and dealt with compassionately by parents

   74. _____

75. Women experience a sexual response cycle which is similar to that of men and can be just as interested in initiating sexual activity as men.

   T. F.

ANSWER KEY

1. T	26. B	51. E
2. T	27. B	52. D
3. D	28. D	53. E
4. T	29. D	54. A
5. T	30. B	55. C
6. D	31. D	56. A
7. B	32. D	57. E
8. B	33. D	58. D
9. A	34. B	59. B
10. D	35. D	60. D
11. C	36. A	61. D
12. T	37. A	62. D
13. B	38. D	63. A
14. C	39. C	64. D
15. D	40. D	65. E
16. T	41. F	66. D
17. T	42. T	67. A
18. T	43. C	68. F
19. F	44. C	69. E
20. D	45. B	70. C
21. D	46. F	71. C
22. F	47. F	72. B
23. C	48. F	73. B
24. D	49. F	74. C
25. T	50. F	75. T

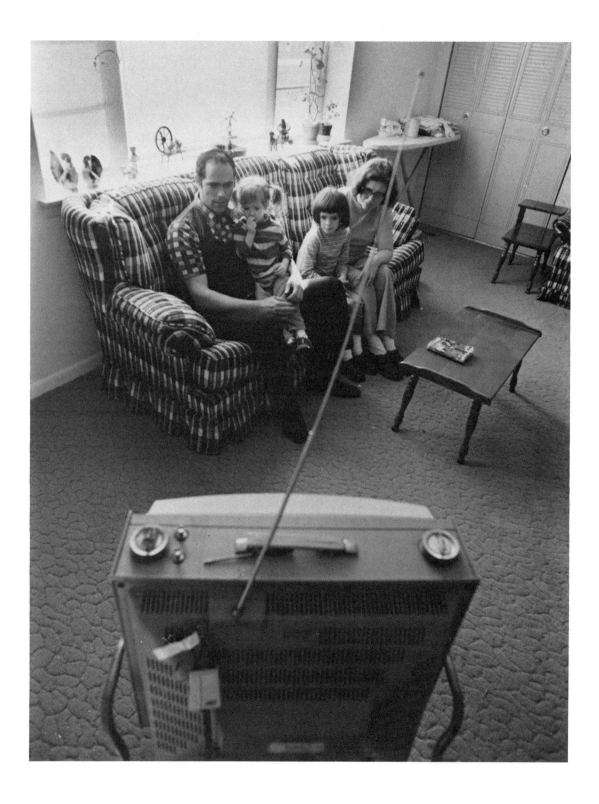

What to Teach Your Children
About Sex on Television

As parents, you are careful with the kinds of food you feed your children, so why are you not choosy about the kind of TV diet your children watch? And make no mistake, our children are watching plenty of television, which is a disturbing fact to most parents. The facts about the impact of television tell us that by the time children graduate from high school, they will have spent 11,000 hours in school and 15,000 hours in front of the television, and that by the age of fifteen the average child has viewed 13,000 violent deaths. Some other statistics to think about include:

- Children spend more time watching TV than any other activity except sleeping.
- Television leads all other traditional influences on our lives (religion was twenty-third out of twenty-four).
- In the average home, the TV set is on for forty-four hours a week.
- The University of Virginia recently reported that among three to five year olds, eighty percent prefer mommy to TV and only fifty-four percent prefer daddy to TV.
- By the time the average child enters kindergarten, he or she has already spent more hours learning about the world from television than the hours one would spend in a college classroom earning a B.A. degree.

These facts point out the primacy of television's influence, yet we seem content to remain indifferent to its potential, its impact, and our power over it. Perhaps we think that by complaining to one another we have done all we can do. We can remain disturbed and frustrated by the appearance of a TV program's images and characterizations that oppose our family values. Or we can better prepare ourselves by taking the responsibility to understand the messages that television communicates every day, twenty-four hours a day. Even the Pope, in the Vatican sex education document, addresses this issue: "There is an urgency that those who are at the receiving end of the media, and especially the young, should learn moderation and discipline in their use of them. They should aim to understand fully what they see, hear and read. They should discuss them with their teachers . . . and should learn to reach correct judgments."

One clear, consistent complaint from most parents is that there is "too much" sex on television. It comes across the screen not in the form of full color close-ups of intercourse, but in subtle "off camera adultery" going on, double meanings, frank talk and "frenzied looks." The point we need to make is that our concern with sex on television does not center on questions about the number of scenes of "actual" intercourse, of shots of exposed female breasts and male behinds. These are trivial questions and they lead, ultimately, to trivial conclusions on the role of television in family life. The more significant questions we need to address are these: What attitudes toward sex and sexuality are promoted by commercial, cable and public television? How do these attitudes shape the values, expectations, and lifestyles of the young? Indeed, how do these attitudes portrayed on the screen affect parents' relationships?

We can best respond by examining the content of television—the images, plots, characterizations, and themes it presents, not only in programming but in commercials. It's a fact that the average viewer, young and old, sees something like one thousand commercials each week. The second concern requires us to probe beyond the particular content of each program, each commercial, to the more subtle layer of unintentional "messages" that television communicates through its structure.

Most parents sadly agree that there is not much new to say about the content of television and the sexual attitudes and values it promotes. What we fail to see are scenes that portray our sexuality as a healthy, positive part of our personality, which is celebrated in homes as part of an intimate, caring and loving relationship. Most sexual encounters on television have a variety of purposes, but the expression of unselfish love, as even just plain, uncomplicated, joyful play, is not among them. Instead, sex is used either as an instrument for profit (watch almost any television commercial) or as a weapon for greater power, wealth, punishment or revenge. All we need to verify this fact is to review any of the critical episodes of "Dallas," "Flamingo Road," "Falcon Crest," "Dynasty" or "Knots Landing."

It's interesting that these distorted messages of sex were supposed to be the result of unhealthy sexual repression and that, as our culture moved toward the full and open acceptance of human sexuality in all its variations, the "seamy" purposes for which sex has historically been used would inevitably decline. Many parents watch these messages on television and confess that we have failed to let go of these negative messages. On the other hand, it seems that as our culture has become more open about sexuality and more liberal in its attitudes, television characters have become more, not less, removed from our traditional attitudes toward sex. It seems that they don't promote respect for all forms of life, the dignity of every person regardless of gender, chastity, and responsible behavior in our sexual relationships. In addition to these distortions of our vision of sexuality, there is a frightening, increasing link on television between sex and violence, especially against women and children. This comes across with the current fascination with such themes as incest, preadolescent prostitution, child molestation, and child pornography.

Ask yourself how many times you have seen prime time commercial television scenes where an adult male and female made love in an apparently caring way. Then think of the number of programs that focus on the theme of rape or threatened rape of young boys, adult males, and adolescent females and the seduction into prostitution or pornography of female and male children and adolescents. Next, consider the commercials in which adolescent girls and children of both sexes either allude to or enact what looks like sexual frenzy, apparently driven by the tightness of their jeans or taste of their toothpaste. Males are portrayed as attaining the epitome of success and power by walking off or driving away with a woman who serves as a sexual door prize.

Cable television fails to bring much relief. A glance through the current television listings reveals that about eighty percent of the cable offerings are masked "sexual situations." It is obvious to most parents that the messages about sex on television are disturbing and contrary to our traditional values. The most significant teaching that television presents is a philosophy which asserts that whatever people want, they deserve to have, and they deserve to have it now. This teaching appears most clearly and consistently within the commercial. For example, "Aren't you hungry for Burger King now?" teases at every hour of the night and day. "Here are your car keys!" "You deserve a break today—so get up and get away!" "You need this car," an ad for a car intones, and a sultry blonde in the front seat whispers, "I really need it," linking the car to a clearly implied need of a different kind. In the symbolic world of the commercial, those who wait between the experience of a need or want and its satisfaction are fools.

The glorification of "whatever people want, they deserve to have it now" is repeated subtly in the very structure of the television commercial. This takes the form of a minidrama in which the protagonist experiences a want as need (girl wants to be kissed by date), encounters frustration (date turns away), is technologically enlightened (roommate gives her Scope), and achieves satisfaction (girl and date fly off to Hawaii)—all in the space of thirty to sixty seconds.

Each commercial takes on the form of a modern morality play that teaches a lesson. As parents and educators of our children's sexual values, there is a revolutionary message on television that we need to challenge. The fundamental principle is that the ungratified need is the major source of human suffering and is, therefore, evil. Another principle is that the source of evil, our "original sin," is ignorance of the techniques or technologies that permit the immediate gratification of our needs. The third principle is that redemption may be achieved instantly, through the acquisition and application of the appropriate technology.

Another way of saying this is that there is no desire that technology cannot satisfy. Therefore, there is no reason to exercise restraint. Eat too much? Try Alka-Seltzer. Too much alcohol give you a headache? Take Anacin. Too much fun in the sun give you a sunburn? Tired eyes? Wrinkled skin? Use Solarcaine, Visine, Oil of Olay.

This philosophy of desire is by no means confined to television. There are exaggerated claims in a variety of advertising mediums. One cannot leaf through *TV Guide*, for example, without coming across a dozen announcements of "technological breakthroughs" that permit one to achieve instant weight loss, instant muscle tone, instant beauty and health without the least sacrifice of one's pleasures. Now you can "eat whatever you like," one ad promises—"pancakes, pastry or pizza, natural food or junk food . . . pasta and ice cream . . . as much as you like"—and still lose weight.

Television presents these sets of values because, more than any other mass medium, it is an integral part of the web of economic relationships that constitute the consumer society. Put simply, the high standard of living we have come to expect requires the constant stimulation of mass production. Mass production requires mass consumption, not only of existing products, but of an ever-increasing variety of new products. To maintain the required level of consumption, people must be persuaded that they need the goods produced and need them now. This is precisely the role of advertising—to stimulate our desire to consume more products. Commercial television stimulates our desires, twenty-four hours a day, seven days a week, fifty-two weeks a year, because its survival depends on advertising.

The economics of commercial television help to explain why the medium places desire and its satisfaction at the top of human priorities. Quite simply, no network can afford to risk the loss of its audience attention, even for a moment. If some need of viewers—visual stimulation, action, excitement, titillation, and novelty—is not instantly met, a simple flick of the wrist may send them and the advertising revenues they represent to another station.

One of the consequences of television's mandate to engage and hold attention is its relentless pursuit of novelty. In a medium that operates around the clock, conventional content is soon exhausted. To satisfy the demands for something new and different, television pushes deeper and deeper into the realms of human experience once considered taboo. On the news or talk shows and interview programs, soap operas, and commercials, no topic is too intimate for exposure to public view. How do the President and his wife handle sleeping arrangements? How does it feel to be raped? How do disabled persons obtain sexual gratification? How do women cope with menstrual problems and men with hemorrhoids? As more and more of what used to be regarded as private goes public, the notion that anything is private begins to disappear. The message that some language and behavior is appropriate for some places and not for others loses its meaning. As a result, the difficulty in teaching our children what is sexually appropriate in certain relationships causes confusion and frustration.

Another message that television teaches is the idea that difficult times have different meanings for interpersonal behavior. Incest is presented alongside beauty hints on morning talk shows, and the difficulties of menopause alongside the stock market report at dinnertime. Except for some early morning evangelizing, the sabbath is indistinguishable from any other day of the week. With the addition of cable and television recording technology, everything is accessible to everybody at any time.

As time and space are woven together, television makes no distinction in personal relationships as well. Traditionally we distinguish among strangers, acquaintances and friends according to the kinds of spaces, times and information we share with them. But television does not respect such distinctions. Strangers reveal the most intimate details of their lives to millions of other strangers, at any hour of the day or night, in bedrooms, kitchens, even bathrooms, without the least regard for the sex, age, or background of the viewers.

As the Nielsen ratings of recent years indicate, there is very little difference in the program preference of adults and children. They are exposed to the same commercials with the same themes; increasingly, they watch at the same times. According to recent surveys, some two million children watch television between midnight and 2:00 A.M. every night of the year. In this context, the fear of some parents that information about sex should be kept away from children seems unrealistic and absurd.

Television communicates messages that rightly distress many parents. How can our young people help but be confused about their sexual feelings, desires, and their expression, when the messages they receive from our homes are so thoroughly contradicted by the messages they receive through a medium as engrossing and compelling as television? How can we help but be confused ourselves?

Haven't many of us internalized the view that since desires are natural, they must be good, and their repression evil, that sin and shame are unhealthy concepts? That, for example, the goal of sex education is the avoidance of unpleasant consequences like venereal disease and unwanted pregnancy? Haven't we come to believe that the withholding of information from the young—the maintenance of adult secrets—is unhealthy and that a reluctance to discuss certain topics in public is a sign of a disordered personality? Have we not already accepted the view that children have the right to be treated as adults, and all adults are equals? But if so, what is our reason for regarding sexual relations between children, as between adults and children, as between consenting strangers, as somehow wrong? Why hedge about sexuality as natural and healthy as our need for eating with special warnings and constraints? If our sole concern is fear of consequences, what answer shall we give to the argument that consequences can always be prevented or eliminated through technology—contraception, abortion, penicillin.

Parents may not know the answers to these questions, but we hope that such questions trouble us. Confusion may be painful, but it is a prerequisite to growth. We need to be at least aware of the contradictions and changes in our attitudes so that we can challenge our young people who have been tremendously influenced by the television medium. Far more frightening than our present distress is the possibility that all of us have learned the lessons of television so subtly, so painlessly, and so well that we stare at the television and wonder what all this fuss is about.

Enriching Family Life
Through Television

Parents know that it isn't normal or healthy for children to sit motionless for three hours. Their minds may be captured by the novelty of television, but their muscles and imaginations are stifled. Often a parent simply has to turn off the set and say, "Go outside and play." Some parents fear the consequences of such aggressive discipline but the alternative is devastating to our children's minds. Watching TV day after day produces the kind of "hypnotic stares" where any suggestion of activity becomes "too much work." The effects of "too much TV" not only interfere with daily routines at home, but with schoolwork as well. Many teachers remark that students resist the usual routine learning skills needed for spelling, math tables, and other basic memory skills. "It's boring" is the usual excuse that students give when their mistakes are pointed out, as if that were a legitimate excuse for refusing to learn personal skills. One simply is not going to learn to write by watching even the most imaginative cartoon on how to write. Television seems to discourage children from sticking to a task because it edits out the dullness of practice, all of the routine necessary to achieve excellence.

In too many homes, communication has broken down completely because parents have allowed television to interfere in their basic need to relate with their children. It's a sad fact that the reason families cannot talk together is because the TV is on. They forget how to talk together, so they watch television, even at meals, so they don't have to talk together. The heavy-viewing family next begins to eliminate other activities. First to go are the walks, picnics, and visits. After that it's entertaining others, ice skating, and days at the beach. All become too much work when there's a set that can be sunk into collectively, at will. Eventually a resentment develops toward anything that intrudes upon television. "We can't come Monday night to adult education because there's football, nor on Tuesday because there's a first-run movie, and so on." Announce the arrival of the in-laws for a visit, and people scream that their calendars are already filled with the need to watch sports, soaps, and sex.

Many parents are concerned about the "hidden" messages of television. We are aware that some programs teach negative messages toward women, children, minorities, and other special groups. Parents are concerned with the desire that television commercials create in their children for toys, junk food, and sex. Also, of course, the evidence of the relationship between sex and violence is deeply disturbing to us all.

But, in fairness, not all television viewing should be considered bad. Television can be a window to the world and reaffirm some of our most cherished values. It can broaden children's knowledge and interests by introducing them to things they've never seen, heard, or done, places they have never been to, people they have never met. Television can also serve as an excellent teaching tool. It can aid in the development of attitudes and behavior patterns we want our children to have. Television, obviously, is here to stay. It is an extraordinary invention that can enrich our children's lives or stunt their growth. It all depends on the choices you have made in guiding their TV viewing in the home.

There is no need to go to the extreme of forbidding any TV viewing in the home. Using television privileges for reward or punishment places too much importance on the medium. You may decide, though, to cut down on how much television your children can watch. Or you may want to be more selective about what they watch. The other extreme is using TV as a babysitter. This can become an easy "crutch" for parents not making an effort to think of something more appropriate. With a little planning and persistence you can change what might be a solitary experience into a chance for family members to learn and draw closer together.

One of the best shows television has produced focusing on the need for parents to talk to their children about sex was a "Gimme a Break" episode where a young girl experienced her first kiss and then later thought she was going to have a baby. The scene further developed as she sought help from her sisters, father, and grandfather, who projected attitudes of uneasiness and guilt. The young girl's reaction to her family's inability to deal with her question is one of anxiety, fear and loneliness. Finally, her tension is noticed by Nell, the housekeeper, who calmly and compassionately asks the girl what's bothering her. The girl pours out her fear while this adult questions the girl as to what really happened. The scene concludes with the adult sitting down with the young girl to read over a book about how babies are made. Although there were some stereotypes presented in the program, such as the inability of the father to talk to his daughter about sex, and the grandfather's lack of interest in sex, still the program contained a number of positive, healthy attitudes that most parents could easily use to teach their own children.

We like to think that television can be used in this way more often. Public television and now cable TV offer outstanding series on great drama, National Geographic specials, and documentaries that have the potential to promote strong, healthy values of people's sexual relationships. But some families never turn to public or educational channels other than to watch the time and temperature, or receive the latest betting results. We do not want to create the impression that public and cable television have the only worthwhile programs. Increasingly, the major networks are sponsoring good drama and specials that provide healthy and wholesome attitudes for family learning, even to the point of showing married couples sharing their love in a caring, not exploitative relationship. We want to offer parents who feel frustrated and helpless by the violence, exploitation, and sexism coming across their TV screen the following guidelines. As parents, we can take back our role as the most influential teachers in our children's values by adopting these guidelines into our homes.

ONE: Watching television gives parents an opportunity to learn what their children are thinking and feeling. It also provides an excellent opportunity to communicate the values and attitudes we want to pass on to our children. In one episode of "Little House on the Prairie," a young girl, about twelve, was feeling attracted to one of the boys in her school. She started to wear her "Sunday" clothes and perfume to make herself more attractive. However, her efforts failed to get her noticed. Instead of being herself, someone who enjoyed playing sports with the rest of the kids, she excluded herself from their games, thinking it was immature and inappropriate behavior for a young woman at her age. Confused, she runs to her mother for advice to learn what people like about her the most. What they had liked was the way she was before wearing fancy dresses or scented perfumes. Mom says, "They like you for who you are." What a beautiful message to share with a young person who doesn't feel very confident about himself or herself. A program like this might communicate the idea that perfume, the right toothpaste, or designer jeans are not the basic ingredients of any healthy relationship. Rather, love and caring are most important. Parents could ask their children questions about how they would feel if their friends abandoned them. Or, even better, we could use the opportunity to share ourselves and our experiences to let our children know that their feelings and ways of thinking are not very much different from ours at their age. Watching programs in this way with our children can frequently lead to family discussions on sexual topics which might otherwise be neglected or postponed.

TWO: To be realistic, no parents have the time to watch television with their children all the time. However, when we are aware of an exceptionally good program that promotes our values, we can make it a priority to watch it with them. After watching the program, another suggestion would be to read a book on the subject of the television special. Visiting the local library can be a great family adventure for everyone to enjoy, including parents. It also should be a part of every family routine to go over the program listings with your child and mutually select programs for family viewing. This time allows you the opportunity to state your limits for television viewing and, most important, to explain your feelings and attitudes regarding the programs. It is easy to find fault with television; much of the programming is poor and mindless. Yet, the fact remains that people get what they want. The choice is still the parents' and with it the responsibility. The primary responsibility for parents is knowing what good programs television has to offer and to patronize these shows.

THREE: A real potential that television offers to enrich family life is to obtain and read the books upon which favorite shows were based. Public television offered an excellent program on the book *How Was I Born?*—a photographic story of reproduction and birth for children by Lennart Nilsson. The value of television is that it can stimulate interest for more knowledge and learning. Children can be encouraged after watching this kind of special to draw, color, make up stories, or act out what they saw on the program. From reading the book, activities or discussions can develop and give us an opportunity to share the correct information they want and need to know.

FOUR: Parents need not limit themselves to only the books on which special programs are based. We may want to know more about conception, fertility, or loving relationships. Parents can take this opportunity to search out other books and articles on the subject, to the advantage of the interest instilled by television. Television's greatest value as a teaching tool is that it can instill a desire to read and learn more.

FIVE: Another teaching method overlooked by parents in using television to enrich family values is to examine programs and commercials with rotten values and sexual myths to teach healthy, positive values and the correct facts about sexuality. We always need good, horrible examples, and they appear often in many of the police stories, talk shows, soap operas, and commercials. Too often, parents allow irresponsible behavior to minority groups, excessive violence and cruelty and exploitation to slip by on the screen without comment.

When heroes are obviously sleeping around, as portrayed by 007, we can wonder aloud why they are portrayed as heroes when they have so little respect for themselves and others. We can get our message across about the need for fidelity, intimacy, and friendship. We do not have to preach, but neither do we have to keep our judgment to ourselves. For example, if one of our children's friends was sitting there, expounding these same values and behaviors, we would probably banish them from our children's circle of friends. Why are we so reluctant to criticize the prime influences? When we are watching a commercial that obviously portrays women as sexual doorprizes or suggests that a particular product can make you instantly popular and attractive, we need to point out the advertiser's real reason for making such incredible statements. We need to offer our children this kind of balance. If your children want to watch a program you think is inappropriate, explain what you don't like about it. Similarly, when a program is supportive of your family's values, you should say so. We need to be gentle but firm in enforcing the family viewing limits. We need to consider the entire family's viewing habits, since dad's need to watch sports can be just as destructive to family life as young people's watching programs with distorted sexual themes that focus on exploitation and violence.

Many of the characteristics and role models presented on television are people whose view of sexuality is negative, guilt-filled, and irresponsible in actions toward others. As parents, we need to provide good role models for our children and young people. Some questions we might discuss with them are: What does it mean to be a man? To be a woman? What kinds of men and women does society need in order to witness to the "good news" of Jesus? These are some important questions for everyone to think about, and for families to talk about together, at the dinner table, in the car, in the evening after homework, on weekends. In this way, children and parents can get closer together because they can learn to talk freely with each other about all sorts of things that need to be discussed, but that are best talked about between people who love and trust one another.

SIX: Another good teaching technique is for parents and children to watch a particular program which deals with some fairly realistic family situations, and then to turn off the set and talk about it. A series like "Fame" is excellent for helping us shape our family values. This series traces the interwoven lives of seven students and four teachers at the School for the Performing Arts in New York City. The students struggle to balance commitments to their crafts with commitments to friends and families. Mr. Shorofsky and Bruno's father tangle about Bruno's readiness to audition for Julliard. Montgomery's superstar mother alienates the whole school by the manner in which she tries to run a school production. When Danny gets his first chance to perform his comedy routines, his father walks out in the middle of his act. Doris befriends a teenage prostitute and tries to get her admitted into the school. Her mother helps her understand that she has not failed this friend when the school refuses to accept her as a student. Just before her solo cello recital, Julie learns that her father will remarry.

The teachers are firm, no-nonsense people who demand and expect excellence from their students. They are not infallible; after Miss Sherwood visits LeRoy's Harlem apartment, she tries to help him by letting him get by too easily in her course. Nor are they pushovers; when LeRoy does not comply with classroom rules, he gets kicked out of the upcoming dance performance. Miss Grant, the dance teacher, does not succumb to the pressure to put him back in the show. In a recent episode, Miss Sherwood faced one of her student's parents about censoring books she has required for her class.

Each student has a unique personality. Each has personal problems as well as those common to all adolescents, from major ones such as drug abuse and sexual experimentation, to the less major such as how to impress a member of the opposite sex, or how to be a friend when you are asked to do something you feel is wrong. The support given each other serves as a model for how people need others to help them achieve their goals.

Television critics have valid concerns. However, we can overlook the potential that a good program has for helping us exercise our values. Programs like "Fame" can jolt our prejudices, trigger self-examination, and assist in the growth of our children.

SEVEN: Watching television together as a family can help us develop our children's taste in television. Just as in reading, the better shows they view, the better the shows they will demand. When a family began watching "All Creatures Great and Small," which was on an educational channel, the oldest teen happened to watch it with his parents. He was hooked immediately and made the comment to the effect that he was unaware there was anything that good on educational television. Now all the children scan the channel's offering along with the others. We need to encourage our children to watch a wide range of programs, besides sports and cartoon specials.

EIGHT: One of the developments of recent technology that has the potential to greatly enrich family life is the personal home computer. It is best understood as the technology of youth. Most teenagers sixteen and younger are familiar with its novelty and potential for learning. Beyond developing skillful hand-eye coordination at drugstores, restaurants, and shopping mall arcades, the excellent teaching tool offers the promise to help end the ignorance in sexual knowledge that plagues our youth today. Programs could easily be developed into software packages containing current and accurate information on sexuality topics. Another advantage of this medium is that when connected to a television set, it provides an environment where young people enjoy learning and can work at their own pace until they understand the material. Programs have the advantage of instantly testing students to see if the material has been learned accurately. This technology will never replace the need for teachers and parents who can help students reflect, clarify, and affirm the values we cherish in our own families. Computer critics need to be heard. However, they often overlook the potential that this technology has for helping us teach the information our children need and want to know. We hope that the novelty this medium certainly provides will not fail to provide the programs our children need to learn.

Another development in media technology is the Video Home System (VHS) which is a new approach to video recording for use in home. Ten million video recorders are already found in homes. They have the capactiy to record and play back programs from your set. A video cassette of the Parents Talk Love retreat is available and produced to serve as an additional educational resource for parents. Like the home computer, the number of programs for video recorders is rapidly growing and their cost decreasing, thereby opening up new potential for sexuality education. Unfortunately, abuses of this medium have already been reported involving child exploitation, which demand that we speak out for the responsible use of this medium which respects the dignity of all people.

NINE: Parents may find television helpful when it occupies the time of children who are sick or who need companionship when parents are working. Television was, and still is, essentially an entertainment medium, although it is gradually becoming more than that. There are times when children need to escape into such entertainment. When parents are away from home or friends are unavailable, television helps to pass a lonely time more quickly. Parents can let their children know that they are available to talk about a program or answer questions. With younger children, we might want to talk about the differences between make-believe and real life, or to discuss television characters and how they are like or unlike real people.

TEN: People need to make a choice regarding the quantity and quality of programs they want their children to view. For most parents, this means taking the responsibility to establish standards in the home. Too often, parents allow unlimited, unmonitored viewing of television. This approach often leads children to acquire many negative and contrary values toward sexuality. Another consequence is "boring" children who are so used to watching television that the suggestion of any creative activity is greeted as "too much work." Also, the novelty of television makes the medium so attractive that the skills necessary for learning, such as patience and persistence, are never developed. Finally, the messages about sexual relationships portrayed in television as a means for power, punishment, manipulation, and violence are directly opposed to the positive, healthy attitudes we want to pass on to our children.

This is the greatest price we pay for allowing our children to watch television without our guidance. Some rules a family might include in their homes are: the set is not put on before breakfast, no TV after school, an hour per day for the eight year old, some shows are not allowed because of the violent or negative messages about family relationships. Again, parents have the choice. We can allow this medium to take control of our families, which leads to chaos and acquiring attitudes opposed to our beliefs and values. Or we can take the responsibility to be selective in using this medium to enrich our family life in positive and healthy ways. The choice is yours.

ELEVEN: Parents do have power to control the quality of programs that are produced for television. The major networks take special interest in letters that either criticize or praise their programs. While we like to stress the positive aspects of television, we cannot ignore its many negative features. Therefore, when you do not like something shown on television, do something about it. Speak or write to your local station, the television network, the local press, your political representative (state and national), your parent-teacher association, or other groups working toward better children's programming. Local groups have often been successful in improving television programming on both a local and national level. At the end of this chapter we have provided the names and addresses of the major networks. Also, we have listed some organizations and newsletters dedicated to promoting better television. It is a good idea to write also to the FCC whenever you send letters to the networks. Parents need to get involved so that television producers, writers, and staff are aware of our family needs and thereby produce the quality shows that can complement our teaching in the home.

TWELVE: An interesting and significant consequence of local cable television is the opportunity to become directly involved in programming. For example, try calling your local cable TV channel, which is often willing to sponsor an educational program of interest to the community. We need to put aside the myth surrounding this medium that only a select few can report, perform, or educate on the TV screen. You can become a producer or commentator, and there is no limit to the good you can do to enrich family life. Your children will want to talk to you again and treat you like a star. Also, this opportunity offers a tremendous potential for teachers to share their experience, skills, and knowledge in sexuality to help parents deal with their children's questions about sex.

Guidelines to Enriching Family Life with the Television Media

1. Watching TV together as a family provides the opportunity for parents to communicate their values.
2. Review the TV program schedule for specials that will enhance your family's life.
3. Encourage your children to read the book that was the source of the story they watched on TV.
4. Suggest other resources on a subject your children have become interested in by watching TV.
5. Use programs, commercials with rotten values and sexual myths to explain positive values and sexual facts.
6. Watch a show that has some realistic family situations and then turn off the set and talk about it.
7. Encourage the family to watch a new educational program for a change of pace.

8. Look for computer programs and video cassette programs as new media resources to teach responsible values and accurate sexual information.
9. Television may be appropriate and helpful when a family member is sick, lonely, or needs companionship.
10. Family viewing needs to agree on set standards, quantity, and quality of programs allowed in the home.
11. Families have the power to control the programs that are produced for TV by writing the networks to protest or praise the programs we watch.
12. Try becoming a producer or commentator yourself. Get involved to insure that TV will enrich your family's life.

Organizations and Newsletters Promoting Better Television

Action for Children's Television (ACT), Quarterly Newsletter, 46 Austin Street, Newtonville, MA 02160.

(ACT) is probably the best-known organization designed to improve what our children are viewing. One of ACT's goals is to educate parents on the uses and abuses of the medium. Broadcasters say that for every letter they get, criticism or praise, they assume there are one hundred other people who feel the same way who have not written. Letters do make an impression.

Project Focus Newsletter, edited by Shirley A. Lieberman. 1061 Broals Avenue, St. Paul, MN 55163.

Clarifies the role, place and impact of television in our lives. "Viewsletter" is published monthly, September through June, and includes articles, addresses and some program reviews.

Better Radio and Television, P.O. Box 43640, Los Angeles, CA 90043.

National Association for Better Broadcasting, 373 N. Western Avenue, Los Angeles, CA 90004.

National Citizens' Committee for Broadcasting, 1028 Connecticut Avenue, Washington, DC 21136.

They publish lists of the most violent and least violent programs and the sponsors of these programs.

Networks

ABC Television Network, 1330 Avenue of the Americas, New York, NY 10019.
CBS Television Network, 51 West 52nd Street, New York, NY 10019.
NBC Television Network, 50 Rockefeller Plaza, New York, NY 10020.

Federal Communications Commission (FCC), 1919 M Street, NW, Washington, DC 20024.

Public Broadcasting Service, 475 L'Enfant Plaza West, SW, Washington, DC 20024.

Everglades Publishing Company, P.O. Drawer Q, Everglades, FL 33939. Publishes TV sponsors' directory.

Questions For Discussion

1. What are some of the programs you presently encourage your children to watch? What are the messages they portray that help to enrich family life?
2. How can parents best prepare to provide guidance in television viewing to their children?
3. How do you feel about your children learning about sex from programs on television? Do you trust this information to be true?
4. What problems can you foresee happening to a child who has unlimited use of the television?
5. Are there any limitations to the television programs your child may watch? Which ones? Why? Who sets the limitations?
6. How do you feel about the use of computers in your home? In what areas do you think they can help your children learn more about their sexuality? How will you do this?
7. Some information that television provides can be greatly increased by using other resources. What are some of the ways you can enrich your child's understanding?
8. How can a parent deal with a child who has been influenced to gain immediate satisfaction of all his or her needs?
9. How many activities outside of television did your family share in the past three months?
10. What are your suggestions to the local networks regarding the quality of its present programs? Are there any changes you would like to recommend? How will you do this?

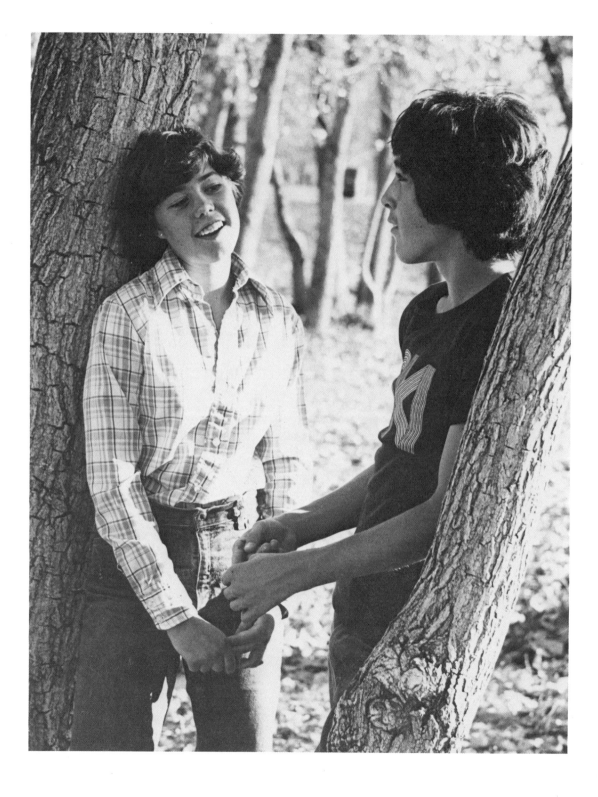

Importance of Intimacy in Sexual Learning

Our ability to experience and nurture intimacy without exploitation in our lives affects our children both directly and indirectly. Divorce, physical abuse, constant arguing and verbal abuse or lack of financial support would seem to hold obvious dangers for children. If negative experiences far outnumber positive experiences in childhood normal, healthy growth to maturity will be unlikely. Children seldom grow to emulate what they do not observe and experience. A person who was never shown kindness will not be kind to others. A child who has only observed and sensed the lack of intimacy, with all its attendant violent symptoms, can hardly grow into an adult who can become genuinely intimate with others, spouse, or friends.

The problem of overt difficulties in parental relationships is easy to identify. We know that children in some families are at obvious risk. But many other children are in much more subtle situations. The prevalence of "good" marriages that last thirty or forty years, "until the children are grown," and then fall apart attests to this. Why do these marriages fail? And what effect do those reasons have on the children over those thirty or forty years?

One of the most frequent statements made when long marriages fail is "We've just grown apart" or "She/he seems like a different person than the one I married." These statements, and indeed the very failure of marriages that once worked, attest to the lack or loss of intimacy, of a true sharing of life between the parents.

Again, its fairly easy to diagnose this problem in the event of divorce. But what of those thirty or forty years previous? And what of all the marriages that continue, nurturing children, living the day-to-day experiences of family life but impoverished of a genuine intimacy between the spouses? What causes this loss or lack of intimacy, and what effect does this have on the children?

There is a story about a woman who was the best real estate agent in her state. She was so good at it that she made more money in her part-time job than her husband who was a lawyer. This didn't bother him at all. Jokingly, he would say he looked forward to her making so much money that he wouldn't have to work ever again. The secret of her success was that she was unfailingly pleasant, patient, and genuinely interested in her clients. But after a while it seemed she was interested only in her clients and sensitive only to them. She didn't have time to hear about her husband's cases or to go to her children's basketball games and plays. She became very touchy and impatient with her family. Finally her oldest daughter said to her, "Hey mom, you've become like bad news. How can you act so charming with your clients but like a total witch to us?" Stunned, the woman took some time off, even made a retreat, and began working on changing her behavior.

This illustrates how we tend to let the important things in life crowd out the essentials. We are shrewd, attentive, careful, persistent, determined, agile, and even, if need be, ruthless in pursuing the important goals of business and profession and lazy and indifferent at pursuing the essential goal of love with our family and God. How does this happen? It takes place gradually. It happens when we are less open and honest in the trivial, minute things, when we let small opportunities pass us by. It happens when we say: "There's always tomorrow. I can't take care of this now."

God is wonderfully merciful, and may give us time at the end of our lives to straighten things out with him and with those we love. But what wonderful opportunities we will have wasted. How will we feel when we look back thirty, forty, or fifty years from today, and see that we have done well in all the important things but have behaved very poorly in loving our families, our neighbors, and God.

The very real, essential, effect of our lives, as parents, on our children's growth as sexual persons is pointed out in the Vatican's document on sex education: "The affection and reciprocal trust which exist in the family are necessary for the harmonious and balanced development of the child right from birth" (n.49). But before many parents can cope with their children's sexual development they first need to heal the wounds of pain, fear, shame, and ignorance which plagued sexual learning in the past. As followers of Christ, our greatest challenge is to allow Christ to heal us. We are called to journey with him to greater health and wholeness. By Christ's personal incarnation he shows us that our goodness as persons includes our bodies as well as our spiritual selves. Parents must realize that we are constantly sending messages about our enfleshed natures to our children. These messages (including sexual messages) may show an adult relationship that is open and playful, with plenty of trust and vitality. Or they may be messages displaying fear, shame, suspicion, disgust, or revulsion with anything involving our sexual natures. One way or the other, messages are constantly being sent. The Vatican document is very aware of this when it says, "A true 'formation' is not limited to the informing of the intellect, but must pay particular attention to the will, to feelings and emotions" (n. 35).

Jesus once said to his disciples: "You have heard the commandment, 'You shall not commit adultery.' What I say to you is: anyone who looks lustfully at a woman has already committed adultery with her in his thoughts" (Mt 5:27–28). In this Jesus is talking about human intimacy. He is not simply condemning divorce. He is opposing the prevalent double standard that imposed punishment on women who committed adultery against their husbands but never found men guilty of adultery against their wives. Jesus was presenting a vision of marriage without divorce because he was interested in transforming the relationship between men and women and eliminating exploitation from that relationship.

In our society, heavily influenced by the media, we have largely lost a sense of the purpose of our sexual natures. We need to relearn that our enfleshed natures draw us to a communion of love with others. Pope John Paul II once said that men ought not even to lust after their own wives. He did not mean that men should not desire their wives sexually or that wives should not desire their husbands. Rather, he meant that men must not dehumanize, depersonalize and treat their wives like sexual objects. He meant the same for women. He was repeating Jesus' message to eliminate all exploitation, divorce included, from our relationships. This opposition to such devaluation is also reinforced by the Vatican guidelines on sex education (n. 28).

As exploitation increases one of the many barriers to intimacy is increased. Who can feel genuinely close to someone they consciously, or subconsciously, feel used by? The most obvious sign that exploitation is rampant in our society is the fact that annually about three millions wives are beaten by their husbands. Sexual assault, within the family, may affect as many as a third of the women in this country. Rape is an epidemic crime, and sexual harassment in the job world and in everyday life is commonplace. However, the marriage contract gives a man no right to force sexual intercourse on his wife and no right to use physical violence against her.

There may be exploitation on the part of wives also. Lacking the physical strength to impose their wills, women long ago learned the techniques of manipulation, ridicule, nagging, and other methods of passive aggression to dominate men. Physical strength on the one hand and psychological cleverness on the other are, if not the stereotypes of husband-wife relationships, frequent enough to seem almost normal.

But not all men and women act this way. Not all men are rapists, not all women are manipulators. Many couples live without this deadly game-playing and lead sexually and emotionally fulfilled lives. Intimacy between husband and wife will only be satisfying when people are able to relate to each other in openness, candor, courtesy, and mutual trust. This is the kind of intimacy Jesus was talking about in the Sermon on the Mount. Sex may come before love, but in the absence of love sexual pleasure rapidly diminishes. Exploitation, manipulation and domination are incompatible with sexual pleasure in any human relationship.

Married spouses have an obligation to each other and to their children to maintain the romantic, erotic, sexually fulfilling dimension of their relationship. They have an even more urgent obligation to maintain honesty, openness, and a genuine appreciation of their partner as a spiritual as well as physical being. A couple's intimacy may grow through genital experiences. It may also grow in a relationship where the partners set aside genital sexual expression. But it cannot grow where one or both partners deny or degrade the sexualness of human nature.

There are many forms of denial and degradation of our sexual goodness. Each one of these acts as a barrier to intimacy. Each one can block the growth of relationship between parents and result in an impoverished environment for children. When children rarely experience their parents' deep affection for one another, how then do they learn to express intimacy, love, and affection for people they will later want as close friends and partners for life?

Some of the barriers to intimacy are very obvious. Others are subtle, creeping into our thought slowly over the years. There is a story of a young couple quietly entertaining family and friends shortly after the arrival of their first child. The guests were alerted when the hostess cried out, "Come quick!" People ran to the baby's room anticipating disaster. The new mother was standing over her new-born's crib beaming. "Everybody look! He's doing something!" She said, "His little face is red!" Getting excited about a baby's bowel movement would seem a bit crazy, but there is something about new life that is fascinating and exciting. The mystery of life is awe-inspiring, and taking care of someone at any stage of growth is a pleasure we often overlook. Instead of enjoying and cherishing our roles as feeders, cuddlers or changers of so many diapers, we tend to grow instead to complain and waste so many opportunities to share the goodness of our bodies. It is especially sad to see how many adults have lost their capacity to enjoy their children as they grow into teenagers. When the wonder and the hugging has stopped, so does the capacity to experience the gift of sexuality. The roles of guardian, provider, disciplinarian and educator, roles that we must fulfill as children grow, often distract us from observing, appreciating, and guiding their growth as sexual persons. Parents are frequently surprised and confused by the realization that their young teens are sexual beings. Fear and apprehension take the place of intimacy, and people call it the "generation gap." Not only does the relationship between teens and parents suffer but the strain on the parents' own intimacy can be tremendous as they cope with this family situation.

A most tragic barrier to sexual and emotional intimacy in marriage is the issue of contraception. Many Catholic women feel trapped in feelings of guilt and shame about their contraceptive decisions. These emotions then prevent them from a fully intimate relationship with their spouse and often prevent them from enjoying intercourse. These women, who have chosen contraceptive methods contrary to the teaching of the Church, desperately need the compassion and understanding of the Christian community. They need to be supported for their decisions, made with tremendous soul-searching and in mature conscience.

It might prove helpful to put this teaching in perspective by reviewing its history. As far as anyone knows Jesus never taught anything explicitly on the issue of birth control. The present Church teaching actually developed over many centuries as it attempted to respond to some of the questions posed by people at various times in history. In the early Christian community, teachers placed emphasis on virginity, often even in the marriage relationship.

As a result of this focus, some strange sects arose who attacked marriage. They taught that marriage, and especially sex, were evil and beneath the dignity of faithful Christians. To respond to these groups, the Church had to answer the question: "If celibacy and virginity are so ideal, how does the Church avoid condemning marriage and procreation?"

St. Paul saw the importance of intimacy as a way of strengthening the marriage bond and, among other things, important for the growth and development of love. Unfortunately, later theologians took a completely different direction. They said that sexual intercourse can be good and holy only when the desire is for a child. The pleasure and joy of physical intimacy is sinful unless the couple clearly desires to conceive children. Another attitude predominant in the first millennium of Church teaching that supported this position was the appeal to "nature." The reproductive system of a person was seen as similar to that of animals. It was believed that animals only copulated in order to reproduce their species. This understanding was completely oblivious to the ways in which human actions are integrated into and bound to the whole personality, physical, emotional, social, and spiritual.

St. Augustine, who died in the year 430, reaffirmed this basic attitude toward sex in his writings. His negative teachings about sexuality dominated the thinking of the Church for many centuries. Pope St. Gregory the Great (590–604) taught that married couples may have intercourse to have children, but if any enjoyment is mixed with it, they sin against the "law of marriage."

These severe attitudes toward marriage and sexuality came under considerable suspicion, not to say disregard through the centuries. The writings of St. Alphonsus Liguori taught a more realistic approach to marriage, stating that married love and affection possess an essential, very primary, significance in sexual intercourse. This essential role of love and affection between husband and wife for intimacy is increasingly emphasized in the teachings of Pope Pius XI, Paul VI, and John Paul II. The recent Vatican statement on "Human Love" says: "Love and fecundity are meanings and values of sexualilty which include and summon each other in turn and cannot therefore be considered as either alternatives or opposites" (n. 32).

The present Catholic teaching on this issue was reaffirmed in the encyclical letter of Pope Paul VI, "Humanae Vitae" (1968), which concluded: "The Church teaches that every act of marriage intercourse must remain open to the transmission of human life."

As Catholic parents we should look to the Church for guidance in coping with this issue. The recent Vatican document states: "Future spouses must know the profound significance of marriage, understood as a union of love for the realization of the couple and for procreation" (n. 61). And: "In order for a married couple to carry out their responsibilities in accord with God's plan it is important that spouses have knowledge of the natural methods of regulating their fertility" (n. 62).

Many Catholic married couples may accept the teaching of the Pope but still find themselves in a dilemma. In their unique family situation, they are involved in what seems to them a conflict of duties—for example, the reconciling of conjugal love and responsible parenthood with the education of children already born and with the health of the mother.

The bishops of Canada in a document prepared to help their people on this issue noted: "In accord with the accepted principles of moral theology, if these persons have tried sincerely but without success to pursue a life of conduct in keeping with the given directories, they may be safely assured that whoever honestly chooses the course which seems right to him does so in good conscience."

The same point was recognized some years earlier by the bishops at Vatican Council II: "This Council realizes that certain conditions often keep couples from arranging their married lives harmoniously, and that they find themselves in circumstances where at least temporarily the size of their families should not be increased. As a result, the faithful exercise of love and the full intimacy of marriage is hard to maintain. But where the intimacy of married life is broken off, its faithfulness can sometimes be imperiled and its quality of fruitfulness ruined, for then the upbringing of children and the courage to accept new ones are both endangered" (*Gaudium et spes*, n. 51).

In the United States the bishops "urge those who have resorted to this never to lose heart, but to continue to take full advantage of the strength which comes from the sacrament of penance and the grace, healing, and peace of the Eucharist."

Perhaps the most grave immorality surrounding this issue is how often this decision is made by women alone, without the loving support and understanding of a concerned spouse. Ideally if a husband and wife have responsibly discussed this issue with a compassionate and informed priest and arrive at a decision based on good faith, then that couple should be assured that they are following correct moral principles.

If a couple cannot, together, come to a decision they are both comfortable with, then the problem may be psychological, not ethical. They cannot scapegoat the Church for their own lack of communication or emotional insecurity or immaturity.

A young mother of five children expressed her anger at being made to feel a failure at Christian motherhood. Her life as a parent was being overwhelmed by children constantly begging for attention, a husband who did not share her concerns about birth control, and a relationship where intercourse made her feel exploited and ashamed. She felt alone, frightened, hurt, and hopeless.

The Church's stand on contraception is meant to be a challenge to marital intimacy. But in the all too frequent cases like this, that challenge has smothered what few sparks of true intimacy there may at one time have been. It has helped to alienate spouses, put an overwhelming burden on women and threatened any further spiritual and emotional growth for the couple.

Both the couple and the Church must share responsibility for breaking down this barrier to intimacy. The Church must be diligent in offering understanding and pastoral counseling and in breaking down the stereotypes that place the burden of decision on the woman. Couples must accept their responsibility for their own emotional growth and seek professional help when the walls begin to grow, not when they are impenetrable. Only with more conscious decisions and action on both sides will marital intimacy and spiritual growth both be fostered by the challenge of responsible contraception.

Another barrier to the growth of intimacy is faced by Catholic single parents. As human persons their need for intimacy is inherent. Yet, without a spouse, they come to some perplexing problems that the Church is only recently beginning to own. These single parents need special support in the caring for children, maintenance and financial support of the home and in overcoming the emotional devastation that frequently accompanies divorce or the death of a spouse. Many single parents have known real depths of intimacy and are now searching to regain or replace it. They may know what they are looking for, though the loss makes the new search more urgent. But, frequently, single parents are just so because of the failure to develop a workable, intimate relationship with a previous spouse or lover. They not only need to find someone, but also to learn the meaning and techniques of emotional as well as physical intimacy. Cynicism is a frequent trap, and, when coupled with feelings of hopelessness and worthlessness, sometimes leads to promiscuous and unfulfilling relationships.

What are the needs that Catholic single people, single parents feel in terms of their sexuality? And how do they satisfy their needs? Of course, the answers to these questions are modified by factors such as age, sex, and previous life experience. Younger singles are more likely to admit the possibility of a sexually intimate relationship in their lives than older ones, and that previously married people feel more strongly the loneliness that single life brings than those who have chosen not to marry.

A single teacher described her life as lonely sometimes, but even married people get lonely at times. Divorced, separated, and widowed persons, on the other hand, touch more often on the deficiencies in their present life: the lack of adult companionship, shared decision-making, someone to talk to, a role model for the children, or someone to share physical comfort with. At the same time they often take pride in their new-found self-sufficiency and independence.

While many single parents eventually begin to search for that one other to fulfill their life, they also need the compassion, support, and intimate friendship of other members of the Christian community. These friendships can and do include pastoral staff, married couples, and even other singles. Many of the needs for child and home care, emotional support, sharing of feelings and experience and just a sense of still belonging to the body of Christ are met in these friendships.

The sexual expression of intimacy through close sexual contact or intercourse becomes a real concern for Catholic singles, especially the divorced or widowed for whom this had been an important and growth-promoting part of their emotional and spiritual lives. The people of the Church must look upon them with compassion, with a willingness to care for them as they search out answers in their lives.

The clergy need to be especially present to these people as they strive to grow closer to the ideals, taking each small step as a slow progression in grace. They need to offer healing, forgiveness and help instead of moralizing and condemnation. Singles can find intimacy in friends, in the community, and, if needed, in lovers, if the Church is willing to be supportive, to accept and acknowledge single parents as an essential part of the people of God.

Family Living as Obstacles to Intimacy

There are two typical ways to cope with the usual distractions, confusion and interruptions in the home. Some parents respond helplessly, screaming: "I can't monitor everything the kids watch on TV. I'm too busy." Parents who react this way spend their lives in constant uncertainty and confusion. They are almost always exhausted, too tired to listen, play or enjoy their families. But living this way has two advantages for the parent. First, parents who allow external forces to control them can argue that they are dispensed from personal responsibility; second, some parents use the excuse that they are breaking their backs to fulfill their role as responsible parents. In such a lifestyle, children are always interfering in a couple's sexual intimacy, but so is everything else. Don't forget to include chronic headaches, in-laws, bills; even choir practice becomes a convenient excuse for the absence of any intimacy. The alternative for coping with the normal interruptions of family life is to establish goals based on values to strengthen and nourish the quality of married love by keeping distractions to a minimum. This requires planning, patience and persistence to live this way along with a sense of self-confidence and self-control.

No parent will ever be completely free from interruptions and distractions in the house. One can choose to dominate and control a hectic life instead of being dominated by it. If a husband and wife say they are too busy with children and career to devote much time and attention to intimacy, then that is the choice they have made, covered up with the disguise of "responsibilities and obligations." Parents should blame themselves for the absence of anything more than casual sex in their marital relationship, not the intrusion of children. The problem is not the intrusion of children into our bedrooms; rather, the real issue is responsible control over the priorities in one's life, such as giving up intimacy to the demands of parenthood. Whether you want to admit it or not, you have made a choice.

Unfortunately, some "Christian" parents fail to inform their children about the importance that physical intimacy has in their marital relationship. It seems that we spend more energy hiding and denying this reality. While modesty and chastity are two primary virtues to be exemplified in the home, scolding a child's curiosity about his or her sexual nature leads to later emotional fears and unnecessary shame as the child develops. In providing guidance, the Vatican document states: "Adults are to be exemplary in their conduct. Christian parents must know that their example represents the most valid contribution in the education of their children" (n. 50).

There are many subtle cues every day as to what a man is and what a woman is, and how they relate to one another. How a family lives its sexuality in the home is crucial to the kind of attitudes children will adopt later in their personal relationships. If the atmosphere of the marriage is frustration, then that is how children will perceive their sexuality. If the marriage reflects a sense of fulfillment and delight, then that is how children will understand the purpose of sexuality. If the intimacy between husband and wife is mutually exciting and fulfilling, the children know it, not explicitly or consciously perhaps, but in their hearts. On the other hand, when parents feel unsatisfied, cheated and angry over a dull or shabby sexual relationship, the children know it too, and this knowledge will have a profound and potentially damaging impact on their sexual development. A woman in her mid-thirties talked about how confused she felt. Married with four children and a husband whom she described as a "good provider," yet she was struggling because the marriage lacked the affection and love so important in the growth of any relationship. She said she couldn't remember ever sitting on her parents' lap. She remarked that there never was any love in that marriage. Yet she desperately wanted a marriage that was full of love, for she had a lot to give. Now, she knew only the pain of loneliness, for her marriage lacked the affection and intimacy necessary for growth.

Children learn correct information, their sexual identity and an appropriate style of relating unselfishly with others from the atmosphere of the sexual relationship between their parents. What other models do they have to imitate? If a child learns that "daddies" are only meant to lie around on the couch to be waited on, to be tough, competitive and unforgiving, and that "mommies" are to be submissive, docile, fragile and sensuous, then that child will find it hard to grow up. On the other hand, from imitating how parents interact, a child can learn that a fully human person is really a mixture of masculine and feminine, aggressive and tender, dominant and submissive characteristics; he or she will come to believe that there is room for risk taking, openness, trust and acceptance. Make no mistake, children learn from the tone of our voices, watching us touch, wink and twist our hips. Our tickling, secret laughter, pat or squeal, our gentle smiles and affectionate touches show children how much we cherish one another.

The best sort of climate for children to mature in is one in which their parents are engaged constantly in "falling in love" with one another—"falling in love" in the sense that spouses are made aware of how wonderful and important they are to their partners. Instead of worrying whether it is fair to the children for parents to devote considerable time and energy to develop their fidelity and intimacy, the moral question is whether it is fair to the children not to. Parents transmit feelings of goodness and acceptance about sexuality to their children almost without realizing it. Children have a natural optimism about all of life, which should include attitudes about their bodies. Parents who encourage attitudes of respect, dignity, and responsibility in sexual relationships give their children a precious gift. However, parents who frustrate that optimism by constantly preaching fear and mistrust of their enfleshed natures deprive their children of one of God's most precious possessions.

A mother who worries over every future possibility and lives a life marked by anxiety and shame creates in her children feelings of timidity and fear. That fear destroys self-confidence and the belief in the basic goodness of others. A father who focuses all his attention on the sexual evils in the world leads his children to see only the seamy side of life and to neglect its joys and promises. Children can grow up in the most rigid and insensitive home climate and achieve sexual maturity to develop a happy relationship in the future—sometimes. But our primary hope is not how a child can survive the mistakes of its parents, but the ideal climate for sexual growth and understanding. Perhaps there is very little a parent does that is more important for his or her children than to share the message that God's precious gift of sexual love brings tremendous happiness, joy, and peace into the life of mom and dad. Parents have accepted this knowledge and exploited this hope for their children. As Christians, it's easy for us to proclaim God's goodness as manifested in a flower, a child's smile, in a grandparent's love for our sons and daughters. Almost everything in God's creation has become a lens through which God's goodness can be seen, has become a "place" where his love can be felt, except in sexual lovemaking. That has usually been considered dangerous, if not actually sinful. Its origin is often mistakenly blamed on original sin, even when it takes place between a husband and wife. A gift of God, a celebration of love and grace? Never!

Most Christian parents have always known, if not in their heads, then in their hearts, how wrong that was. Their experience of their sexual intimacy helped to bind them together more closely to increase their joy in their union. It actually gave them strength to meet the difficulties of marriage, parenting, friendship, and daily obligations with greater patience and love. How, then, could it be dangerous, much less sinful? How could it be anything less than an opportunity for grace, a time to experience a warmth and care so extraordinary that its root must be traced back to God's love for them? This is the future we should want our children to hope for in their sexual awakening.

Some parents make the mistake of condemning sexual behavior so strongly that they inflict attitudes of disgust and shame whenever the topic of sex is brought up in the home. Rather than project an image of a wrathful God who will crush them for any sexual thoughts and fantasies, we need to instill virtues of chastity, modesty, respect, and responsibility in dealing with our sexual lives. Some parents make the mistake of feeling that they are responsible for everything their children are and everything they do.

They even try to live their lives for them. All that should be expected of parents is that they do their best for their children. While parents cannot live their children's lives for them, they can try to set good examples without trying to masquerade as perfect. They can try to pass on to their children, as opportunities arise, the standards and values by which they live. The children can think about these standards, experiment with them, reject them, return to them, discuss them with others. All this helps young people mature.

In addition, children will inevitably look outside the family for information, opinions, and experiences whether we want them to or not. We recognize that television, friends, books, and magazines are reaching them in their homes constantly. Parents cannot and should not try to isolate their children from these outside influences, although they can provide help to select the experiences their children will have. The main goal of parents is to help their children equip themselves with information, reason about facts, be aware of the wonder and beauty of the "good news" about their sexuality and have an openness and understanding to be available for them.

Young people need an interpretation of their sexuality more than anyone else precisely because they have just discovered it. Sexual rebellion and experimentation among teenagers are, in fact, a search for meaning. To put it another way, if it is clear that the parents have obtained great enjoyment and satisfaction from their own sexual relationship, the children are perfectly willing and eager to find out what their values are, how they managed when so many have failed. If, on the other hand, it is clear to the children that their parents don't make love all that often and don't enjoy it that much when they do, there doesn't seem to be any reason why they should listen to their parents telling them what is right and what is wrong. It is that simple. All the rules, lectures, warnings, and temper tantrums in the world are no substitute for a mother and father who obviously enjoy going to their bedroom every night.

Parents have been so close-mouthed about sexual lovemaking, about the need for intimacy and friendship, that they have been duped into suspecting there is indeed something dangerous and sinful about these things. As a result, sex has been too often taken over by those who degrade it and use it simply to make themselves rich, or, worse yet, wish to project their fears on children. They will not cease either until perhaps they can no longer be heard in the crowd of voices from parents who understand and celebrate the gift of sexuality and prove that when God looked over "all" that he had made and proclaimed it very good (Gen 1:31), he wasn't kidding.

We cannot deny or wish to belittle the confusion and anxiety in the sexual lives of young people. One of the main reasons for the confusion is that only a few young people grow up in a positive, healthy, loving sexual climate created in their home by involved and prepared parents. The challenge is to live family life aware of and affirming our sexual gifts and not in constant worry and chaos. This is our greatest and most difficult responsibility. Parents must not fool themselves by delegating the task to the schools, teachers, nuns, priests, neighbors, grandparents, or television.

Today the Church is encouraging parents to take back control of their children's education in sexual learning. And single parents are capable of providing competent guidance. All parents must show perseverance, tolerance and patience. The best parents are those whose physical relationships reflect a deep friendship, a close bond of respect and love for one another as persons. The goodness of sexuality and enfleshed bodies will be caught by children living in this kind of home climate. The solution to dealing with children's sexuality is to eliminate those obstacles which keep parents from being at ease with their own sexuality.

Questions for Discussion

1. Depending on your particular lifestyle, how would you describe your sexual feelings, attitudes, and the "climate" of sexuality in your home?
2. How do you think your children perceive your attitudes toward sex?
3. What obstacles, if any, hinder "intimacy" in your home?
4. What areas in your life do you think you need to take greater responsibility and control of in order to better enjoy intimacy in your relationship?
5. How do you open a discussion about "intimacy" with your spouse?
6. What areas of growth in "intimacy" would you like to develop?
7. In what ways do you perceive the Church's teaching affirming your need for sexual intimacy?

8. What messages about your sexual relationship do you want to pass on to your children?
9. What are some of your fears regarding your children's sexuality?
10. What issues in sexuality would you like your pastoral community to deal with in the future?

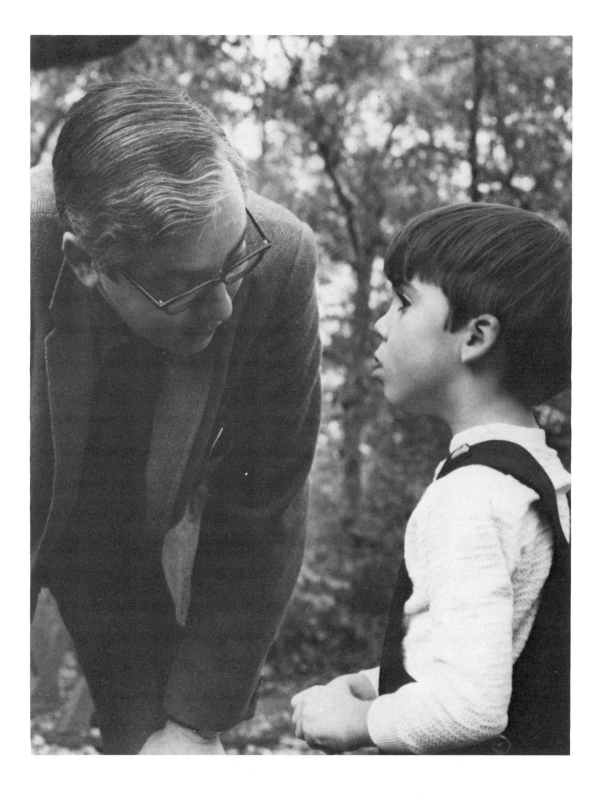

Talking About Sex

This entire book is a preparation for talking about sex. In this chapter, we want to bring to the fore some more specific preparations and guides for conversations about sexuality with your children and with other adults. It is nearly impossible to converse in an area where one has no knowledge, attitudes, or values. So, when a conversation about sexuality, one of the most intimate, mysterious and vital facets of our lives, arises, all of our past knowledge, experiences, attitudes and values are brought to our attention. These elements are what we will draw upon when it is our turn to speak. But these are often disturbing to us. Many of our experiences have not been helpful or pleasant. Our knowledge may have large gaps which make us uncomfortable and insecure. Our attitudes are often those of people who are searching, yearning, hurt, embittered, twisted by earlier experiences, or discouraged, and our values are frequently questionable. All of these things pour into our hearts and minds when we are truly required to say something meaningful about our humanity and sexuality.

Ah, but you say we talk about sex all the time, and it is not as dramatic as all that. It is true that television offers us sexual situations every evening and all day too. Talk shows, magazines, radio, records, and everyday casual conversations zero in on the latest sexual information, sexual fads, behaviors, and misbehaviors. Sex and sex talk seem to surround us and everyone takes it casually. But most of these things don't really touch us; they don't call on our heart to respond. We can be casual in a sexual conversation. We can tell jokes, glamorize, exaggerate, cover our ignorance with popular myths, hide our real selves. We do this often. It's a skill that children begin to develop in their early teens. But do we always want to hide ourselves? Don't we want to give our real selves to our children? Don't we want to be truly intimate with our spouse? Don't we want to be genuine with our close friends? These are the most meaningful yet often fearful relationships of our lives. They can be deep and growth-filled, which takes some effort, some risk. Or they can be superficial, safe, and full of loneliness.

When we prepare ourselves to talk about sexuality, we must be willing to take those same risks of self-disclosure and openness that are required in the other deepest facets of our lives—love, faith, and friendship. This risk-taking is usually a difficult thing at first. Few of us are really taught or encouraged to do this as we grow from infancy to adulthood. This is normal. Such risk-taking was difficult for most of our parents. *Talking* about sexual matters was almost impossible for people of our parents' generation. Instead they joked, even though they faced almost all the same life complications we do. They lived with the history and traditions passed to them from their parents. We've already seen how negative attitudes about our bodies and their normal functions crept into our religious thought. The social customs of the Victorian age, whose roots reach back into the "courtly love" ideas of the Middle Ages, along with romanticism, highlighted the religious misconceptions and made an exaggerated and distorted sense of modesty the social norm. Somehow, in passing along mysteries from generation to generation, we often convey the fear and distress of them without their fineness, beauty and naturalness. Add to this the lack of biological information, with the fear and shame that usually accompany ignorance, and we begin to sense the atmosphere surrounding sexuality that our great-grandparents, grandparents, and parents, with all good intentions, couldn't help but pass on to us.

Today, impersonal sexual conversation is much more open and common. Recent scientific discovery and the legitimizing of the serious scientific study of sexuality in its own right, combined with the ruthless drive of the media to gain our attention and dollars by exposing every aspect of life to scrutiny and sensationalism, have created a truly uncomfortable situation for people who were raised knowing only the secretness of sexuality. They find it difficult to hold sacred something so open and well-studied. Transition is often painful, and adds a new dimension to the problem. Those who embrace the new openness eagerly are viewed with suspicion. Old values and attitudes of respect seem to have gone down the drain of time, leaving many stranded and bewildered.

So we come to speak of our sexuality with a foundation of cultural and religious difficulty. However, we must still add another burden. We each have our own personal history which causes us to be shy in sexual matters. Our own body image, begun in infancy; our earliest learning, when scolded for playing doctor or slapped for masturbating; the outrageous myths of our early teen years; the shame and guilt of our first sexual experiences; the pain of negative adult experiences—all these come to haunt us as we join or initiate a conversation about sex. It's difficult to put these aside, impossible to ignore them.

The very first step in talking about sex to our children, or to other adults, is to come to grips with our religious and cultural history, our own personal history, and our need to risk disclosing the deepest parts of ourselves. We must come to grips with the fact that this just is not easy. And that's O.K. It doesn't have to be easy, and we need not be embarrassed any longer by our common history of uneasiness. But neither should we be satisfied with it. A beginning must be made somewhere. In beginning to talk about sex, we must never forget our values and attitudes, where we got them, and how we want to pass them on to our children and others.

Beginning, Young Children

The most natural people to talk to about sex should be our parents or spouses. But since it's often almost impossible to initiate a conversation with parents after a lifetime of silence, and many are divorced or separated, though this book is focused primarily for parents, we'll begin with the easiest people to talk to: the very young ones.

Not everyone would agree that it is so easy to talk to young children about anything in the adult world, let alone sex. Many adults find little children cute and cuddly to hold, needing teaching, care, and frequent scoldings, but not conversation. Many adults think they are talking *with* little children when they are really talking *at* them. Many people think that little children don't really understand much of anything. But they are wrong. Children are striving to understand everything. There is the whole of life in this world to talk and learn about. Pre-school children are listening and learning all the time. They may not learn quite what we intended, and they do not possess the polished thought processes of adults. They are children, and just as their bodies, though recognizably human and with all the basic human needs and functions, will need years of development to adulthood, so too their minds are in many ways similar to those of adults but must go through a long process of development of thought and understanding. Children must build both a process and a technique for thinking and analyzing, as well as a storehouse of sound information and a history of experiences before they step into adult thought. This is why it is so easy to talk to little children about sexuality. They don't have all the emotional, cultural, religious baggage that we do. Most pre-school sexual conversations are pretty simple and straightforward. "What's that?" (pointing to a penis on a statue) is a clear-cut question. No shame, no guilt, no long discussion of women's lib, premarital sex, or the morality of sculpturing is requested—simply a name for a body part. If parents can say, casually, "That's a penis," understanding what the child needs to know, then two things have been communicated. First, that's a penis (fact). Second, there is no big deal. Mom or dad will answer questions, and the child can trust that mom or dad will fulfill her natural needs, in this case the need for information.

With young children, the first communication about sexuality is sometimes unspoken—a cuddle, an expression, the tone of voice, who plays how with baby, mom or dad? As communication becomes verbal, body parts are normally the main topic of conversation. Parents reading this book, if they have young children, have a great chance to begin talking about sex with an ease and grace that many others have passed up. "That's your scrotum, that's your nipple, that's your penis, that's your vulva." How simple! Baby isn't going to respond with shock, horror, or embarrassment. Baby will love every word you utter in a loving, warm, and matter of fact tone of voice. Baby will have started to like himself or herself, and you've started talking about sex.

For practice, just try saying a string of words, you and your child's other parent, or a friend: "coffee, tea, vulva, ear, knee, milk, breast, scrotum, butcher, lamb chops, clitoris, belly button, apples, homosexual, opera singer, heterosexual, education, masturbation . . ." Don't die laughing. It's good for you!

Admittedly, it doesn't stay this easy for very long. But the next stage is not insurmountable. The child who asks "What's that?" (the penis) may then want to know: "What's it for?" Steady, parents—the pre-schooler is not interested in the mechanics of intercourse, but rather wants to know about how boys and girls are different. Well, of course all boys have a penis, and all girls have a vulva and a vagina. Sounds simple, doesn't it? And, if you've passed stage one, it's not too hard to say that either. This child may carry on the conversation to ask about other familiar boys or girls or family members. Or the child may remark about the size and shape of the penis, the color of the statue, why the statue had no clothes on, why he or she has to wear clothes, or a hundred other turns the mind may associate with this experience. This all depends on what the child has seen and learned in the past about your attitudes and willingness to answer anything. We can't possibly walk down each of these paths with you in this book, but we can remind you to remember all that's inside you when you take that deep breath before answering. Certainly Uncle Frank, the president, the basketball coach, the store clerk, and even the Pope, as of today, all have penises, because all are male. Why be nervous about saying so? "Admit" it with reluctance in an embarrassed tone and you've taught that something about our bodies is shameful, and it's not chins and knees either. Admit it eagerly, joyfully, with a smile and a twinkle in your eye, and you have taught that our bodies are beautiful, wonderful, even if mysterious creations. Don't be dismayed if the child laughs and compares the penis to any number of other familiar objects—worms, sausages, etc. This association, which would perhaps be vulgar coming from an adult, is a normal and healthy part of childhood thought. (Possibly the vulgarity of it in adults lies only in its immaturity.)

As young children learn to ask questions, their parents must learn to ask questions too. Childhood thinking is somewhat different from that of adults, so children are often misunderstood. Children often drop statements or questions at which their parents drop their jaws. Parents who have truly realized that children don't have the same wealth of experience and knowledge and attitudes they do are a step ahead in this phase. The pre-schooler who proudly announces that she was "playing doctor" may not be implying the same idea that pops into Mom's or Dad's head at hearing the phrase. Nor does the child, boy or girl, who says, "I'm going to have a baby," or "I got screwed by Joey," or a thousand other seemingly scandalous things. Here it is that parents should question carefully and casually. "Did you have fun playing house, honey? What did you do?" is much more helpful to the child and parent than "Oh my God!" The child can then respond with what actually took place. Was it simply playing roles, or was there some real physical exploration going on? If it was the former, the conversation will go in other directions. If it was the latter, then the parent may wish to continue casual questioning to find out just what the child learned. Explanations of how improper this behavior is should not be given to pre-schoolers. You can say something like this: "All little boys and girls want to know how other little boys and girls are made. I certainly did. But once you know because you've seen it, you don't have to go on doing the same things. Remember, we all like privacy, and these are all part of our *private* lives." Period. It is a normal part of their growth process. With children older than six years, parents will have to make a judgment, depending on the child's response to family values. If the child is genuinely lacking in biological knowledge, now is the time to remedy this. If the children fall into this play out of boredom, new activities can be found. If an older child is influencing a younger one, they can be interested in separate activities. It is important to be able to see the situation through the children's eyes. This is done best by giving the child a chance to explain. Then gentle action can be taken based on adult wisdom.

Simple questioning, however, should never resemble and feel like an interrogation. Children are perceptive and will not continue to be open when they feel pressured or manipulated. An anxiously-phrased question can make a child immediately guilty and fearful. Parents should strive for truthful communication when they question and not subtly pronounce judgment, or strip the child of privacy and self respect. Often the words of the question betray the purpose:

Tommy: "Where did I come from?"
Mom: "I told you last week—from Buffalo. Don't you remember? Why do you want to know again?"

Tommy probably won't want to ask more about babies; he feels pretty dumb for forgetting last week's conversation already. Or the tone of voice.

Tommy: "Where did I come from?"
Mom: "Do you mean what city or country? Or was there something else you meant?"

This lets the child know that there is another meaning for "come from" besides location. He'll continue to ask more since Mom seems to imply it's O.K. to ask.

Sometimes the pattern of questions could be changed, according to what feels natural. Some explanation could precede the question:

Mary: "Why do boys wear only shorts on the beach, and girls have to wear tops and bottoms?"
Mom: "Because that's one of our social customs. Other places in the world have other customs. Why are you interested?"

In this way the child is not frustrated that no information is forthcoming. The answer is there. But mom also gets a chance to find out what the child is thinking and keep the air open for continued exploration of customs, roles and responsible behavior.

Often a parent will feel no need to question or "check out" what's going on in the child's mind. But the parent who does so often enough to keep in touch with the child, to let the child not feel threatened by a question, is setting a valuable foundation. In later years the question may become a more valuable tool for parents to keep their sanity as their children's questions and statements become more complex.

Another key factor in talking about sexual matters with small children is the art of being simple but truthful. Some parents think that to give an explanation a child can understand means "baby talk" or "fairy tales." Nothing could be further from the truth. "The stork brought you" is not only cruelly dishonest, but the vocabulary and concepts are no easier for a three year old to understand than "You grew inside mommy." Granted, the child cannot yet quite grasp "grow," but suppose that he or she wants to know where the stork got him or her from?

Telling the truth, in simple but correct terms, on a level of understanding the child is prepared for, is probably the one greatest commandment of talking to children about sex—or anything. This follows from the technique of careful questioning. Children themselves can let you know what they are prepared to understand, if you're willing to ask and listen closely. In the section on child development we talked about how a child's ability to understand the reproductive process progresses through several stages before being mechanically correct. By checking with children you can find out at what stage they are and answer their questions and tolerate their lack of adult reasoning with patience. Children who do not yet understand the idea of growth certainly do not need a discussion of the male seed and the female egg. They just won't comprehend it. It won't hurt them because it just won't register in their train of thought at all. But a child can be told, "You came out of a special place in Mommy because we love you." Vocabulary and attitudes should be included as well as process information. Urine, vulva, scrotum, uterus are not difficult words. Their truthfulness adds much to a healthy attitude. Children who have never heard anything but wee wee and piss will much later find out that urine is an uncomfortable word to say. Why become uncomfortable about something everybody does all the time and doctors always ask about?

Speaking the truth, simply, is a skill that takes time to develop. It involves understanding the information to be given as well as what the child needs to know. Neither of these is beyond the average parent. Here are four year old Mary and Mom dusting furniture together:

Mary: "Linda said that babies come out like poop."

Mom: "You mean bowel movement? How does she know that?"

Mary: "Yeah, her big sister told her."

Mom: "Well, dear, I think her big sister might have made a mistake. Do you know how babies come out?

Mary: "They come out through your bottom?"

Mom: "Not exactly. There's a special place where babies grow called the uterus. And there's a special passage for babies to come out through called the vagina, which is not the same as the anus, which is where bowel movements come out. Babies really have nothing at all to do with bowel movements. Do you see what I mean?"

Mary: "Yes, babies aren't like bowel movements; they're people."

This conversation is casual, and Mary feels free to open up the idea to her mother. Though it's not exactly a question, she is looking for information just the same. Mom checks things out a bit to find out what Mary already knows and what she needs to know now. Mary hasn't asked about the pain of childbirth or hospitals or anything else. She wants to know about places and the relationship between bowel movements and birth. So, to a four year old, mother doesn't go into the details of birth. She clears up the misconception Mary has now. Her answer is truthful, contains some vocabulary and sticks to what Mary wants to know. At the end, mother rechecks to see if Mary has grasped the idea correctly. Mary's answer to this is really not clear. Mother may want to mention the words uterus and vagina again to help the girl learn them. This conversation could continue if mother senses that Mary is interested in more information; more likely, it will end for now and be picked up again some hours, weeks, or months later. At age four, Mary still has lots of time left to learn these things and mother need not be in a hurry. To have begun is enough for now.

The setting is important in conversations about sexuality, too, along with time of day and the normal rhythms of family life. Sexual conversations should be kept casual and within the regular activities of the family. While doing household chores together, parents and children can talk naturally. Driving to the store or to school or to grandma's house provides a captive audience for both parent and child. Mealtimes may be ideal if the family is used to eating together and sharing conversation. Parents should not feel that a sexual question must be answered in the bedroom with the door closed. This conveys attitudes of shame and guilt that should be avoided.

Occasionally a child's question comes at a time or place that is very awkward for the parent—in a busy supermarket, when Aunt Prudence is over for tea, when the boss and his wife are visiting, or when the parent is just too busy or upset by something else to answer. Parents should feel that it's O.K. to (very occasionally) put off a child's question until a later time. But this needs to be done gently and honestly, and the parent *must* provide an answer to the child's concern as soon as possible, as promised. If this happens only infrequently, and if the parents are truly sincere and the child's needs are met, there should be no ill-effects on the child's willingness to ask more questions. Children easily learn that sex conversations at the store, school, or maybe even grandma's are out of place and inappropriate. This is not harmful so long as conversations *do* take place at home or where it *is* appropriate.

A common fear of parents before imparting sexual information is: "What if I make a mistake?" We all make mistakes, and we all manage to recover from them. Mistakes are a part of life. They can sometimes be very growth-producing. Fear of mistakes should not paralyze us.

Parents often fear that they will mistakenly tell a child too much. If they learn to question carefully to discover what the child wants and needs to know, this won't happen. If a child knows enough to ask about something, then the child is old enough for the answer. Also, information that is a little advanced for children will probably go right over their heads, or not be interesting enough to be thought about or remembered. This kind of "telling too much" refers to answering children's questions and giving correct and wholesome sexual information and attitudes by reasonable adults. We have occasionally been criticized with the example that, surely, taking a child to an X-rated movie must be harmful, and that this is certainly telling the child too much. This criticism is quite irrelevant because X-rated movies, scary stories, and passionate descriptions of scenes of intercourse were never meant to be educational experiences, not for children. They have their own positive or negative functions for adults only, and obviously are not what was meant by telling a child too much. The fact still remains that to give a brief, simple, truthful description of sexual intercourse (the man puts his penis into the woman's vagina and ejaculates sperm) to a child who is old enough to ask is not harmful. It will not make the child any more likely to try this activity. It will not make the child fearful of sexuality if it is told with an attitude that conveys its beauty and goodness. If the child really wanted to know something else, and the parent gave the description of intercourse, that's O.K. Either the child will understand it and appreciate the information, or he or she will let it pass, perhaps catching a phrase here and there to ask about some other time when it becomes important.

Another fear of "mistakes" comes when parents find that, without thinking, they let slip a real blooper of misinformation. Children will learn completely and independently that adults make mistakes. We can't hide this from them. So it is best to maintain their trust in us by admitting our mistakes. Perhaps the second hardest phrase for many of us to say is, "I made a mistake" (the first is, of course, "I'm sorry"). But what power to join and heal this phrase has. If you tell a child something incorrect, out of ignorance or thoughtlessness, you should correct it. The child may later have access to the right information. But wouldn't you rather it be you who tells the truth and is looked up to as honest and caring? Children adore and respect adults who can say cheerfully, "Guess what. I made an awful mistake the other day," and then go on to give the right information.

Sometimes children ask for answers we just don't know. So tell the truth: "I don't know, but I'll go find out." If you have a book handy, all the better. Parent and child can look for answers together. But if this isn't possible, then find out as soon as possible and return to share the new knowledge. No one is expected to know everything or to have every answer on the tip of the tongue. The most important thing in communicating about sexuality is to be willing to learn and to share. It is not important to be all-knowing.

One more concern many parents have about their pre-school children and sexual knowledge is what their children learn from others or are telling to others. What they are hearing from neighborhood playmates can be easily discovered by gentle and casual questioning. If the information is correct, so much the better; you can confirm it and be glad to know there are other parents nearby who are doing a good job. If the information is false, then it can be corrected just like any other mistake and it has served to open up a new conversation. Parents are sometimes more uncomfortable with the idea of their children educating the neighborhood. But think—why shouldn't they be? If what they are saying is true and good, who should deny its being shared? Parents may fear gossip and reprisal from their neighbors. When this happens, remind them that it is the truth that sets us free, not fairy tales and fear. Ask them if they expect you to tell lies to your child. This may not always be a simple situation, but then we must act on our beliefs. Our own children will respect us for this and model themselves after us.

In working through how to talk to young children about sex, we've discussed several main points which are rather basic and should follow through into all other age groups.

First, assess what the child wants and needs to know, and speak on a level that the child can understand. Second, tell the truth; don't be afraid to say "I don't know" or to look things up. Third, tell just enough. Let the child ask for more. Fourth, check up often on what the child is absorbing; this keeps the lines of communcation open. Fifth, don't preach or scold when asked for information. Respect the child's need to know. Sixth, be true to your values and attitudes. Make these clear to your child; reinforce the goodness and joy of human sexuality as our Creator gave it to us.

School-Aged Children
Through the Pre-Teen Years

Talking to a "middle aged" child can cause parents a bit more concern. These children have many more sources of information besides their parents. Their questions need more complex answers—biological, relational, and moral. Peers begin to influence these children. Their school may have a good sex education curriculum, a poor sex education curriculum, or none at all. Parents who have grown in communication with their children through the pre-school years have a headstart. Parents who haven't can, with a little work, still catch up.

The same general guides about sexual communication hold true as with younger children. However, the idea of telling the truth simply will probably often cause the most difficulty for parents. As children's questions become more complex their answers must also become more complex. Parents now need to try their hand at giving complex information in both facts and attitudes, in terms clear and simple enough for their children to understand. Nine year old Tommy has heard the other kids on the bus talking.

Tommy: "Dad, why is it wrong to say 'fuck you'?"
Dad: "Do you know what the word 'fuck' really means, Tom?"
Tommy: "Yes, well, I guess it has something to do with making love—doesn't it?"
Dad: "Yes, some people use that word when they mean sexual intercourse. When people say 'fuck you,' do they sound very loving?"
Tommy: "Gee, no."
Dad: "That's what's wrong. It takes something beautiful and good and makes it into something nasty, used to hurt people."

In this conversation, Dad has tried to deal with the complex issue of sexual slang, the human inclination to use intimacy to hurt those at whom they are angry. This is a complex issue and it is to be hoped that their discussion will continue as Tommy encounters slang more and more.

After nine or ten year old Tommy's first experience of an X-rated film on cable TV while staying overnight with a less supervised friend, a conversation like this might take place.

Tommy: "Why do people like to have sexual intercourse?"

Mom: "Because to love each other and have beautiful body feelings as well as emotional feelings about each other is a great gift given to men and women by God."

Tommy: "But it seems so yucky."

Mom: "For people who don't love each other, perhaps it is yucky. Intercourse is truly beautiful between people who love each other enough to be married. It's really right and very good only between people who love each other very much."

Tommy: "Oh . . ."

Mom: "Sometimes when we just see something, we don't appreciate it. Do you think the actors in the movie really loved each other?"

Tommy: "Probably not."

Mom: "That's right. And so maybe that's why it seems yucky to you—it wasn't really right."

Premarital and extramarital intercourse and X-rated movies are complex issues even for adults. Yet Tommy needed to work out some attitudes concerning both the goodness of the sexual act and why some movies are not approved by his family. Mom did not hit him with an ultimatum, "The Church says . . ." or, even worse, "God says . . ." or "You rotten kid—you shouldn't talk about that." Rather, she tried to simplify the complex for him. She assured him that intercourse is good, that it should be special. She led him to understand why the movie made him feel uncomfortable about an aspect of love he had always been taught was good.

This conversation is surely not perfect, and in your family, it might go quite differently. That's O.K. We don't want you to memorize our answers, as that wouldn't be being true to yourself. You might emphasize how sexual intercourse is private between two people and that someone watching can never fully appreciate it, is not sharing the love, and so really is not right. You might emphasize the importance of the marriage bond and of fidelity and commitment. These are all good things, but don't try to do them all at once. Remember the age and mental capacity of the child. A pre-teen does not yet understand the intense emotional and physical responses which are involved in sexual intercourse, nor is he fully able to grasp the moral aspects. You'll have plenty of time to discuss these in later years when they are relevant to the child. For now, concentrate on responding to the child's need.

As children move through the early school and pre-teen years, the influence on them of people outside the family increases continually. This can have several effects on communication about sexuality within the home. At first, information and misinformation will both increase.

Eight year old Mary is watching her father fix the lawnmower:

Mary: "Linda (her eight year old friend) says it's bad to watch her baby brother get his diapers changed. But sometimes she peeks when her mom does it."

Dad: "Oh?" (He's a little thrown off . . . is this important or just chatter?)

Mary: "Yeah, she said next time I visit I can peek with her."

Dad: "What do you think her mother will say?"

Mary: "Oh, Linda does it all the time, I guess it will be O.K."

Dad: "Why do you think Linda's mother said she couldn't watch?"

Mary: "Because girls aren't supposed to see boys undressed. It's bad."

Dad: "Is that what you think about seeing boys undressed?"

This is a complicated topic. Dad has to deal with several things. He wants Mary to have a good attitude about bodies. He doesn't want her to think it's bad to see a baby boy undressed. But he wants her to respect the customs that other families have in their homes, and he wants her to continue to be friends with Linda, yet respect the authority of Linda's mom. In the conversation above, he is still just figuring out the situation. It could continue something like this:

Dad: "You know, Mary, each family does things a little differently, has some different customs and different rules. I guess Linda's mom has her own reasons for Linda not to come into the room while the baby is being changed. But in our family, we really don't think it's wrong to see a baby undressed. Babies are quite beautiful. Remember when we visited Aunt Helen?"

Mary: "Yeah, I helped give cousin Eddie a bath. It was fun. It was really funny when he wet all over Aunt Helen."

Dad: "Yes, it is funny when babies do that." (They both laugh.) You know, Mary, our bodies are beautiful gifts from God, and as we grow up, part of appreciating that beauty is to be modest and keep some parts of our bodies covered in public."

Mary: "Yeah—that's like wearing a bathing suit at the beach, but not in the bathtub."

Dad: "Right. But with babies, most people are so happy that baby has a healthy body that modesty isn't important yet. So when you visit Linda again, you must do what her mother asks. Peeking is not nice if she doesn't want you to. Maybe you and Linda could find something more exciting to do?"

Mary: "Maybe. I think she has Pac Man now. I really like that."

Again, this is not a perfect conversation, but almost none are. Mary and Linda will probably peek again. But dad has laid the groundwork. He has let Mary know what his attitudes about bodies and modesty are, and also how he feels about the authority of other parents, and the customs of other homes. If this conversation is backed up by others and by other positive activities in the home, then Mary won't pick up negative attitudes about nudity inappropriate to their own family's beliefs.

Can you pick out some of the techniques dad used in this conversation? A casual style and setting . . . checking out what this child needs . . . making his own values and attitudes stand out . . . a bit of teaching . . . keep ideas simple, on the eight year old's level . . . a touch of humor never hurts . . . keeping communication open.

Other effects of the common increase of sources of sexual conversation outside the home are experimentation with bad language, sexual slang, sexual jokes, and an attitude of degradation toward some aspects of sexuality. This happens slowly, gradually as the child's experiences broaden to include a large number of public toilets and older children on the school bus and in the neighborhood. A parent may not even be aware of these at first. Some children are more vocal than others. Some are shy and some share more of their experiences with their families.

In one family, a fourth grade child had been on a school outing where children of several grades were on the bus. During part of the trip she had listened to some older boys talking about a particular misdeed and how later they would be punished if caught. That evening at dinner she related how the boys were probably "going to get screwed" for what they had done. With these words came silence at the table. The message was clear that something bad had been said; however, exactly what it was just wasn't made clear. The girl felt embarrassment and shame. Eventually the conversation picked up along other topics.

This is an example of "unconversation" about sexual slang. The idea that it was bad came across pretty clearly. But some other negative things came with it. The child suffered loss of self-esteem for simply not knowing that the word was unacceptable in her family. Perhaps she would have difficulty asking any further questions about sexual slang. For quite a long time to come, she might have a very foggy idea about just why sexual slang was wrong. She missed out on some positive reinforcement of the goodness of sexuality.

The slang in this example is quite mild. Children can, and usually do, bring home much worse. School-age children through pre-teens usually learn the classical, well-worn words first. As teens, they will later get into the really hot expressions as their rising sexual tensions seek release. Parents should take an active part in dealing with this situation. But first they must come to grips with sexual slang for themselves.

Some adults are very sensitive to sexual slang—so much so that the sight or sound of these words disturbs them to the point of being quite beyond clear thinking. Other adults may be nearly immune to these same words. The reasons for both situations are many and complex, but parents at both extremes, as well as those in between, need to examine and perhaps reset their attitudes toward sexual slang so they can best help their children.

In the Parents Talk Love Retreat there is an activity where parents write down all the slang words they can think of for various body parts and activities. "Elbow" never has more than one slang synonym. Others, such as penis, breasts, menstruation, and intercourse, always have a dozen or more each. Why? Elbows seem to have no outstanding interest or excitement about them. Children all learn what an elbow is without any particular fanfare. But of course sexual words carry much more emotional impact. This emotional power lends itself to several uses. Sexual slang words may be used to shock, control, or put down others. They are often used in an abusive and hurtful way. In some groups, sexual slang helps a member "belong" or shows how "tough" the person is. It draws attention and recognition, either positive from peers or negative from parents or those in authority. Sexual slang is sometimes used in ignorance; the technically correct words just aren't known, or are too unfamiliar to use comfortably. Last, but not least, sexual slang may be used out of long habit.

If we examine more closely the kinds of language available we find four basic modes of expression. Scientific or correct language is well defined and precise; the meanings are quite standard. Urine and urinate have exact meanings for anyone who knows the words. Society has developed a set of "common" or "polite" terms. These are euphemisms, which beat a word around the bush on their meaning. "Go to the bathroom," "duty calls" and "powder my nose" are attempts to say it without really saying it. This is another hilarious throwback to our Victorian past. Children understandably have a bit of difficulty with this charade when they are very young. They are too honest when speaking. Yet many parents obviously don't think their children can or should use the scientific or polite terms, so we end up with even more ambiguous phrases like "wee wee," "number one" and "I have to make bubbles." From all of this confusion, pre-teen, teen and adult slang has its birth. With the secretiveness, the ignorance, and the ambiguity comes the emotional impact and power of these same words.

So, what to do about this situation? The first and most difficult task for parents is to become desensitized, then resensitized to these words. When a nine year old shouts "fuck you," or a six year old says "boobs," or a spouse says "cunt," the adult must be able to defuse the power of the word, bypass the emotional shock wave, to deal with the person and the feelings behind the word. Shock, horror and disgust have no place here and don't help solve anything. One can't help others if one is too caught up in one's own emotion. The parent who wants to really help a child with the twin problems of bad language and dirty jokes must be able to cope with hearing these without falling to pieces. The next step is to become resensitized. Clarify for yourself why these words are not a part of your vocabulary or that of your family's. Be very clear on these reasons. Be able to defend them without undue emotional upset, but defend them nonetheless. Become sensitive to the real and harmful effects of these words and expressions. Be prepared to explain clearly how the use of sexual slang dehumanizes the nature of both men and women, both the users and those it is used against.

Again, when talking about the use of sexual slang with your family, it is important to defuse the word, to take part of the mystery and secretiveness out of it by saying it yourself. Sometimes children really don't know the meaning of a particular word. This meaning should be made clear, as should your feelings about it.

Dad is playing basketball with eleven year old Tommy and his friend Joe. Joe bumps into Tommy.

Tom: "You fag, Joe. Watch out."

Joe: "You watch out yourself."

Dad: "Whoa, fellas, that kind of talk doesn't go over big on this team." (The boys stop playing and look a little shy)

Dad: "Do you know what that word means, Tom?"

Tom: "Yeah, I guess it means you're gay or queer."

Dad: "What does that mean?"

Tom: "Well, homosexual, I guess."

Dad: "Do you remember when we talked about that a couple of weeks ago?"

Tom: "Yeah."

Dad: "So, Joe must be a homosexual. How did you decide that?"

Tom: (embarrassed) "Well, no, I guess I didn't mean to say that."

Dad: "Well, Tommy, we need to say what we mean. Otherwise how will we understand each other? What did you really want to say?"

Tom: "I was mad 'cause he ran into me."

Dad: "Good. It's O.K. to be mad. But say just that. When you're angry, say 'I'm angry.' O.K.? Don't hurt people with words you don't mean."

Tom: "Yeah, Dad. O.K."

In this conversation, Dad comes on very strong. Some parents can't pull this off. It would be too embarrassing for the child to be scolded in front of a friend. But in this situation, Tom and his dad have a history of real communication, and it can be done in a good-humored way. This also provides a bit of education for Joe, who witnesses the exchange between father and son. In other homes, this talk could take place after Joe goes home, when parent and child can be alone together.

Focusing on the high degree of emotion involved in slang expressions brings us to the next area of communication about sexuality: emotions. Understanding and communicating our emotions does not come naturally at any age. The success or failure of many adult relationships rests on the partners' ability to identify, deal with, and communicate their feelings effectively. This skill needs to be learned. Very young children can be helped to identify when they are angry or happy or sad. If parents accept all these feelings as normal parts of being human and don't take personal offense every time a child is angry or sad, then they can help their children grow in emotional health.

A key rule in talking about emotion at any age is not to deny or minimize the emotions of the other. For example, five year old Bobby's pet hamster has died.

Bobby: (crying) "Do you think Blinky will go to heaven?"

Mom: "Don't be stupid. Hamsters don't go to heaven. I don't know why you're making such a fuss; it was just a hamster."

Bobby: "But I miss him."

Mom: "Only babies cry over dead hamsters. Now go outside and have a good time playing with your cousins."

In this conversation, mom is devastating Bobby, adding scorn to his broken heart. There are many possible results. Bobby may learn to keep his emotions to himself, and he may become a target for later ulcers and high blood pressure. One of the surest pathways to intimacy and understanding, the sharing of grief, is being closed off. Bobby's feeling of self-worth are undermined. His maturity is questioned. His own sense of caring and compassion is being turned around to hurt and insult him. Undoubtedly, many children experience episodes like this at times. Parents are busy, under stress, or stricken by the same grief that affects their children. If these unfortunate conversations are few and far between, and if there are enough positive experiences to outweigh them, the child may eventually struggle toward healthy, emotional maturity. But if these are the norm, then no doubt the child will have chronic emotional problems.

How do we help the mid-years child toward growing emotional health? Use casual conversations, perhaps while watching TV, or at meals, to identify a wide range of emotions, and give names to them. Find opportunities to discuss the differences between emotion and how a person acts on that emotion. Accept the child's changing moods. Help the child to identify the feeling and decide what to do about it. Let children see you dealing with emotions, accepting them, but not acting on them without conscious choice.

Eight year old Patty is playing with her two year old baby brother who, in play, bites her. Dad is watching TV.

Patty: "Hey, you rotten kid . . ." (she raises her hand to slap him).
Dad: "Hold on, Patty! What's the matter?"
Patty: "He bit me. It hurts."
Dad: "It looks like you're gonna hit him."
Patty: "Yeah, he hurt me."
Dad: "I know it hurts, but please don't hit him. Then you'll both hurt. Would that make your hand feel better?"
Patty: "No . . . but he isn't supposed to bite."
Dad: "That's right, but he'll have to be a little older to understand that. Now come here and let me kiss where it hurts."

In an example, more to our topic, Bobby is twelve. He has been quiet all through dinner.

Mom: "Bobby, you kind of look as though you don't feel too happy."
Bobby: "No, I don't."
Mom: "Can you tell me what's wrong?"
Bobby: "Well . . . what if you sort of like someone and she doesn't like you, if she does mean things to you?"
Mom: "You're feeling kind of hurt about something someone did to you at school?"
Bobby: "Yeah. It's nothing." (He's embarrassed to tell.)
Mom: "We often get hurt by other people's words or actions. It's okay to feel bad about it. But can't I help you figure it out?"
Bobby: "It's Donna. I try to be nice to her, but she's always doing stupid things to me. Today she scribbled on my math paper."
Mom: "Do you think she likes you and that's the only way she can get your attention?"
Bobby: "No, she always does mean things."
Mom: "I guess it's pretty hard when you like someone and, no matter what you do, that person just doesn't like you back."
Bobby: "Yeah."
Mom: "It must make you feel sad."
Bobby: "Will people ever like me? Girls, I mean?"

Mom: "I'm pretty sure they will, Bobby. You're a neat person, you know, and when they discover what they've been missing, why you'll have girls all over the place. Just give it a little time. Kids don't always see each other very clearly when they first begin to grow up."

It has taken mom quite a bit of patient acceptance of Bobby's feelings before the real problems come out. Emotions are often more difficult to talk about than other things. Mom has let Bobby know his emotions are okay and normal. She's helped him to identify why he feels badly. He's afraid that girls will never like him, self-doubts that we all share. Mom could have repeated this a little more clearly at the end, but she does try to teach a bit about early adolescence. Many people would throw out the phrase, "Give it a little time," as a put off. If that's a parent's standard answer, "Just wait till you grow up," it *is* a put off. Used occasionally, and when it's really true, kids can understand that there are some difficulties they have because of their age. They can understand that there is hope for change and that part of this change is time. It helps take the burden off them personally, and places it on all of us, through our development.

The increase in the need for biological knowledge during the grade school years is altogether a different cup of tea. It often throws parents for a real loop. Most parents received very little physiological training when they were young, and so feel hopelessly ignorant in this realm. We've suggested before that parents who wish to bone up on their sexual biology should get a book intended for teenagers and read it. These usually include most of the basic information, and they are readable and interesting. Another good idea is to have a book on family sexuality available in the home. When biology questions come up, parents can then feel secure that when they've reached their own knowledge limit, help is close at hand. The pictures and diagrams in these books not only help to illustrate descriptions that parents have already given, but give the "O.K." to looking for sexual information in well-written books by responsible and knowledgeable writers.

Probably the most difficult aspect of conversations concerning sexual biology is being comfortable about saying, "I don't know." Parents need not feel any loss of respect for not being walking anatomy texts. By the time children have had a few months of organized education in a public or private school, they become quite comfortable with our repository of knowledge—books. If parents begin when children are young and act as though checking out information in books is normal and respectable, their children will benefit in two ways. First, they will probably learn more accurate information than they would have without the books. Second, they will develop an attitude and habit of using books as tools. So they get not only information but the skill to find more information whenever it is needed, throughout a long future.

A last important aspect of sexual conversation in the school age and pre-teen years is the parents' interaction with the child's school. As we said before, a few schools have good sex education programs, more have mediocre or abbreviated programs, and about ninety percent have nothing at all. As a parent you may wish to ask about the program your child will be a part of. You may ask to see curricula (course outlines) and materials, and ask about how the teachers are trained. Positive, supportive parental involvement neither means parents who sit back and criticize everything nor parents who say "yes" to anything. If your school has a sex education program, perhaps you could become involved in some way in improving its effectiveness. Teachers are often glad to have help in searching out new materials for their classes. Parents can be invaluable in developing training evenings for other parents so that all can keep up with what the children are learning. The possibilities for positive help are endless. If your school has no organized sexuality education curriculum, or relies heavily on the "locker room talk," or one week of the health curriculum, then perhaps you could become involved in forming a sex education curriculum committee. In school districts with heavy parental participation, sex education courses are generally well-planned, well-monitored, and comprehensive. Controversies are solved with little trouble in these districts because the parents are already fully involved in the program.

Another aspect of parental involvement in school sex education comes to the fore when a particular problem involving the child or the teacher arises. This will require some real communication on the part of parents. Perhaps a teacher mistakenly passes along some misinformation, or voices an attitude that is contradictory to those of the home. The parent should carefully question the child to be absolutely sure of what was said. Next, the parent should be very clear that he or she has correct information and balanced, rational attitudes. The next step is to talk to the teacher. Make an appointment to talk in person. Many an angry phone call or note has been made on impulse and regretted later. In talking to a teacher about a particular topic, the parent should remain calm and open-minded. Perhaps the teacher had good reasons for what transpired. In a conversation like this, all the rules for an adult talking to a child still hold true. Both parties should come through with self-respect and reputations intact. Some education should happen. Some checking-out, questioning and stating of personal values should take place. It should end with both people feeling that they have benefited from the experience.

These conversations may be long; adult attention span is typically longer than that of children. Here is an abbreviated example. Ms. T. is a sixth grade teacher in a Catholic school, and Mrs. R. is a concerned parent. They have already talked for a while and have looked over some films and materials:

Mrs. R.: "Now tell me how you teach about homosexuals."

Ms. T.: "This topic does not come into our curriculum in a formal way until the eighth grade, so I would not introduce it to the sixth grade children as a planned lesson. However, if they were to ask about it in class, or if it came out in some other context, I would tell them what the Church teaches—that we must be compassionate and not condemn."

Mrs. R.: "But, you know, the Bible strictly condemns homosexuals, and I don't want my daughter to think this is a choice for her. I want her to know that this is wrong, that these people are sinners."

Ms. T.: "Yes, no parents want their child to be a homosexual, but, you know, this is not something people choose. The reasons for homosexual orientation are just not known. What we do know is that none of these children will have to choose, but that a few will *discover* that they are homosexual, whether they want to be or not. The Church urges us to be compassionate toward these people, to offer them Jesus' love and acceptance.

This conversation could (and did) go on for quite some time. The parent needed to air some feelings and also to learn some information. The teacher tried to be gentle in teaching because she was well aware of the history from which this and other parents have come. It was good for the teacher to hear about the parent's fears and concerns. The teacher would spend extra time and care when this topic came up in class.

If a parent talks calmly with a teacher and still is not satisfied, the next stage is to go to the principal of the school, not to the coffee klatch! Keep the problem where it belongs. Be rational, and don't make a community issue out of a private misunderstanding. Neither you nor your children nor your community benefits from an uproar with no positive outcome.

Talking to Teenagers and Young Adults

All too often parents say little or nothing about sexuality to their children until they enter their teen years, and the need becomes overwhelmingly obvious. These parents tend to rely upon either the "big talk" or an argumentative approach. It should be clear by now why the "big talk" doesn't work. The information that any person can absorb at one time is limited. What is of most interest, and therefore of most importance to a particular teen, will change from one day to the next. So the "big talk" probably contains too little and too much information. A large portion of it will be irrelevant. It will probably be uncomfortable and embarrassing for both the parent and child and therefore somewhat destructive of positive attitudes and good family relationships.

So the big talk is out, but so is the crisis-oriented or argumentative method as well. In the crisis approach, nothing is said until there is a problem. When mother is horrified at what she finds in Tommy's room, then she says a piece of her mind about sexuality. Or when Mary lets slip that she went to an X-rated movie with her girlfriends, dad blows his top and goes into a moral lecture at the dinner table. These ways of talking about sexuality reduce this whole broad aspect of our personhood to nothing but a problem, to be dealt with only in angry, fearful situations. Interest in their sexuality then becomes something that young people learn to hide from their parents. They develop feelings of shame and fear. They are denied accurate information and they become open to exploitation by many elements of our society.

But it doesn't have to be that way. Parents who have talked with their children from the time they were young have to make adjustments as the children grow into their teens. They have to learn to let go, to let their actions do much of the talking, to be firm in their beliefs while understanding that teens need to change and risk. These parents will be living this out on a foundation of communication. Though there will be times of bewilderment, they will ultimately know and understand their child, who will know and understand them as parents.

But what of those families who haven't yet built such a foundation of communication? Can they ever really catch up? The hard fact is that they can never recreate a history that is already past. Many professionals feel that to begin talking about sexuality to an already-teen is simply putting a bandaid on a problem. Teens have already learned a good deal about their parents, simply by observation over the years. They have begun to develop their own personal histories. They have seen the values their parents have lived out, and they have surely absorbed at least some of them. But other values may have been lost just because they weren't made clear or weren't explained when the child saw the need for them. Questions that went unanswered or conversations that were aborted at the first feeling of discomfort all have left their impressions. The teen has already learned a great deal about sexuality, much of it negative.

Whole books have been written about communicating with your teens. Here we offer just a few basic ideas. But we believe that there is always hope for communication. The teen's greatest need is for his or her parents' love and time. Time is the best place to start as it is the most obvious; for to refuse or fail to spend your time with your child is to devalue that child. Expressing genuine love is growing difficult in epidemic proportions in our society. At least time can be counted and measured. If you have not built a foundation of communication with your children as they've grown, if you've inherited teens through divorce and remarriage or adoption, whatever the reason, start spending time with them now. Arrange for activities where one or both parents can be together with the teen for some period of time without other family members demanding your attention. Make this an activity that is not distasteful for the teen and where your full attention can be spent on the teen. Make these times short at first, then increase them as you both become more comfortable.

Everything in life takes time, so learning to communicate with teens will also take time. Don't come on like gangbusters from the start. No one of any age likes to be trampled by someone else's ideas, opinions or feelings. Do a lot of listening, not just hearing words, but genuine listening to the thoughts and emotions of the teen. You may be surprised and pleased at some of the things that come across. Remember what stage the teen is at emotionally and developmentally. Remember the teen's need to test and try rules, to take risks, to pull away from family and become an individual. You can't develop a new relationship with a teen without some knowledge, self control, and reflection on your part.

Teens who have had negative experiences with family or authority will very naturally resist new offers of friendship. They will need to be shown with great gentleness, over a long period of time, your concern for them. Some may never respond. Some have already turned completely and with finality to their peers for information and attitudes about sexuality, so they may view anything you say simply as an attempt to control them. Truth, integrity, and example are the only alternatives here. Teens are extremely sensitive to hypocrisy in adults. "Do as I say, not as I do" is the worst of all attitudes to present them with.

Even teens who have not had particularly negative experiences in the past may not necessarily be a piece of cake either. It is the nature of the teen to be somewhat at odds with parent and authority. When we accept this as normal, we can begin to deal with it as gracefully as possible. The kinds of affection children responded to eagerly when young will often be met with embarrassment by teens. This shakes adults' self-image. ("Am I a bad parent after all?") It shakes their sexual self-image. ("How can I be woman-mother or man-father to this person now?") Teens call their parents to grow into new people, to show affection in new ways. Most of us are very fearful of these changes in ourselves, especially when there are sexual implications.

The possibility of sexuality-based problems in teens is another cause of anxiety and so becomes a wet blanket on conversations with them. An alarming number of teens impregnate or become pregnant in our modern society. No parents want this to happen to their child. But somehow it does happen, and this causes fear in parents. Some teens will realize that they are homosexual and will try to hide it from their parents. Others will drop it like a bomb, leaving parents in a state of panic or numb. Most parents don't fear this in their teens as directly as they do pregnancy or venereal disease, but it all adds up to a plague of parental uneasiness with teens and sex. So whether you've been talking about sexuality with your children from the time they were young, or you've married into or adopted a teen, or have just avoided most sexual conversation in the past, teens present new challenges to parents who want to help them with knowledge and attitudes about sexuality.

Many of the techniques helpful in talking to teens about sex are extensions of those used with younger children (or adults for that matter). Checking out, asking questions to determine what the teen already knows and needs to know now, is invaluable. But it must be done carefully, not as interrogation or prying. Teens are very sensitive about their privacy. They should be respected in this, but parents still need to have a continuing knowledge of their children's progress. Sincerity in questions comes not so much in the words said as the tone of voice, the expression, the history of the parents' integrity and concern.

Truthfulness is, of course, fundamental, but it takes on a new dimension as teens' needs and questions become different from those of younger children. Teens who did not get accurate biological information may still ask questions along those lines. But the majority of questions will now center on behaviors and values. The teens are beginning to prepare themselves for adult decisions. They may ask how parents feel about some topic or what the parents did when they were young, or what they would do now. These are the most frightening and difficult questions to answer at all, much less truthfully.

Seventeen year old Mary and her mom are driving home from the grocery store. They have been talking about the dating activities of some of Mary's friends:

Mary: "Everyone knows Larry and Kathy are going to bed together. But I guess it's O.K. because everyone knows they're going to get married anyhow."

Mom: "They're going to get married at eighteen?"

Mary: "Oh probably not until after college, but someday for sure."

Mom: "What will they do if she gets pregnant?"

Mary: "Well they must be using something . . . you know . . . to prevent that."

Mom: "Did they say so?"

Mary: "Not exactly, but everyone does. Didn't you before you were married?"

So, mom was going along easily, checking out to see what Mary was thinking about contraception. Then the boom fell. The truth may be easy or hard. If mom is totally against contraception, never used it, was a virgin when she married, and lives out those values to this day, she can affirm them truthfully but gently. She doesn't want to condemn Mary by condemning her friends.

Mom: "No, as a matter of fact I didn't. Your father and I believed very strongly that it was God's will that we be virgins when we married. So I didn't need any contraceptives."

Mary: "But wasn't it hard? I mean, it's normal to have sex, isn't it?"

Mom: "Of course it was hard. But that's what I believe. It means a lot to me to live by my faith."

Again, mom is not condemning, but gently and firmly standing up for what she believes. Right now she doesn't want to argue about the normalcy of premarital intercourse. She wants to answer truthfully about her own values. This conversation could go differently if mom lived her values differently.

Mary: "Didn't you before you were married?"

Mom: "You know, I felt very bad about it, but I did. I had to hide it from my parents, and I wasn't really sure I was right. It was an awfully hard decision for me, and sometimes I wish I had made the other choice."

Mary: (surprised) "Why?"

Mom: "I was afraid that your father wouldn't love me enough to get married, and we almost didn't. I wasn't living by the values I had been taught. It spoiled a lot of things that might have been nicer for us."

In this answer, mom is trying to be truthful about the tension and guilt that often come with hard decisions. She wants to tell her whole story, not just give a simple "yes" that could mean many things.

These are not the only possibilities. The answers may be as infinite as the people answering. Parents today have varying attitudes about contraception. They have dealt with Church teaching and conscience in a variety of ways. Their teens need help in processing this balance in their lives. What parents tell teens will only be helpful if it is genuine, from the heart.

There may be times when the whole truth is too difficult or inappropriate to tell. Nineteen year old Ted is helping dad paint the garage. Ted has been away at college and is feeling very mature:

Ted: "Gee, dad, when you got divorced, wasn't it hard not having sex and all?"

Dad: "You know, Ted, that was a very upsetting time for me. It's so personal that I don't really feel comfortable talking about it. Maybe some other time, after I've had more time to think about it. O.K.?"

Ted: "Sure, dad. I didn't mean to hurt your feelings."

Dad does not want to talk with Ted about his sex life, and he is honest enough to say it. But he does so gently, respecting Ted's feelings and desire to be close to his dad. Not wishing to talk about something with a teen is certainly legitimate. But it should happen very infrequently or the teen will quickly pick up the message and go elsewhere for information and attitudes.

In seeking to tell the truth to teens, we may have to search for these truths when they aren't clear to us. This can be a disturbing process. We may not have found these truths when we were teens. We may be living in compromise, in ambiguity, or in the dark concerning some questions. So when our teenagers demand answers, we are put on the defensive. We want to try to avoid this feeling of being personally cornered or attacked, not by rejecting the teen or the question, but more by accepting the fact that none of us are perfect, none of us have all the answers. It's too easy to turn this feeling of personal frustration against the teenager who is already irritating us in other ways.

In talking with teens about sexual matters, their intense emotional involvements and responses are often hard to cope with. Teens are susceptible to the whole range of adult emotions. Increased hormone and energy levels and the newness of these emotions can bring them out with a frequency and intensity that is startling to adults and a source of turmoil to many teens. Talking about these emotions can help young people keep their footing. They can be helped to realize that this is an important and normal part of growing up. They can learn to "flow with" many of these strong emotions without necessarily acting on them. They can practice appropriate expression of many emotions, particularly anger and "love." Teenage "love" can be anything from an intense pleasure in chewing a particular gum, to appreciating a certain rock band, to respect and loyalty to the school basketball team, to affection and familial love for a baby sister, or to a strong, physical, sexual response to another teen. A really important role of sexual-based conversations between parents and teens should be slowly to sort out these emotions, to identify levels of liking, loyalty, affection, respect, and love. Often it is not clear to parents just what constitutes genuine love. This may become a mutual research project. Why date a particular partner? What characteristics are most important in a date? Why go steady? What are the differences between selfishness and affection that is generous and self-giving? How to reconcile concern and self-giving with the strong physical desires of the young? How to know when love will last? How to survive a love that has dissolved? Tough questions, indeed. Adults have difficulty with these. Yet we expect many teens to work through them on their own. These are not topics a parent can just bring up, point blank, over the dinner table with the other parent reading the paper and the six year old making castles with her mashed potatoes. Parents need a terrible awareness of teen needs. They need to be on their toes, present in mind and emotion when their teen is ready for their help.

Mom is washing the dinner dishes. Sixteen year old Stacy is passing through the kitchen with her school books, ready to settle down to homework.

Mom: "Say, Stacy, how is Patrick? We haven't seen him in over a week. He must be awfully busy."

This isn't an essential conversation, so mom is going to leave it open to see if Stacy will want to talk.

Stacy: "I don't know. I don't think he's that busy. He just hasn't been around."
Mom: "I thought you were pretty good friends."
Stacy: "Yeah, but I think he's really mad at me now."
Mom: "Oh? Why?"
Stacy: "Well, I've been spending a lot of time with Chip, you know, the football captain."
Mom: "That's nice, the football captain. Do you like him?"
Stacy: "He's O.K. Sometimes he does some goofy things. But all the girls think he's really gorgeous, and maybe I can get him to take me to the sophomore dance."

Aha! It takes a little time, but there it is. How to decide between one who is a friend and one who is "goofy" but prestigious? Now this is not yet a crisis situation. At this time, Stacy is not sexually involved. As a high school sophomore she is not thinking about life commitments just yet. But she is learning about friendships, relationships and integrity. Mom will not try to force or even push her. But she will try to help Stacy see what is going on.

Mom: "Don't the other girls think much of Patrick?"
Stacy: "I guess they all get along with him all right. Why?"
Mom: "I was just trying to think for myself what the difference between Patrick and Chip might be."
Stacy: "Well, Chip, he's the greatest! He's the captain and all the guys know him. All the girls wish they could go out with him."
Mom: "Does he go out with lots of girls?"
Stacy: "Oh, all the time. But now maybe he'll just go out with me!"
Mom: "Do you think you'll go out with him just to impress the other girls?"
Stacy: "Huh?"
Mom: "I mean do you really want their approval so much that you'll risk not really having a good time just to look good?"
Stacy: "Why do you say that?"
Mom: "Well, you said Chip was kind of goofy. It sounds like you don't really like him that much. What if you don't get along?"
Stacy: "Hmmm—I never thought of it that way."

Now, this is not a particularly earth-shattering conversation. But mom is sowing the seeds for later conversations. She is sensitizing Stacy to what might really be happening. But she is not making a "big deal" out of it, so she leaves Stacy to think about her situation. Stacy will make her own decision about whether to go out with Chip or not. It seems she probably will. He may prove to be the kind of person she likes, or maybe not. Either way, mom has helped her to be a little more conscious of her motives for decisions about personal relationships. It takes many of these little conversations and many experiences and failures to develop genuine integrity in relationships. This is not earth-shaking, just one small step along the way.

With teens, another kind of conversation often develops which is not as casual and easygoing as those we've shown thus far. These are teens' heated conversations concerning conflict situations. They revolve around a difference of opinion or values between the parent and teenager, and often break into arguments and even "fights," verbal or physical. The "fight" and argument part should be avoided, for in these both teens and adults tend to lose sight of their real goals. The only goal usual to an argument is to win, and the real issue may be completely forgotten in the heat of battle, in the drawing out of all sorts of emotional ammunition and positioning for power.

When a genuine conflict arises between parent and teen, it is the parents' responsibility to keep the real goals in sight, to keep the conversation away from the battlefield, and to set the tone and open the doors for genuine two-way communication. The teen's natural need to develop a personal strength, separate from parents, and test their own choices is often stronger than their ability to view the situation objectively. Old emotional issues, bad habits, and continuing family irritations should be strictly kept out of a conflict conversation. Whether a young teen goes to an unchaperoned party or not has nothing to do with whether he keeps his bedroom picked up or treats his younger sister well. An older teen's decision to use contraceptives has nothing to do with whether she smashed up the family car when she was learning to drive, or is failing in school. Keep the conversation on the issue at hand; do not drag in other issues.

In typical conflicts, parents have two basic goals: to influence the adolescent's behavior, and to impart their own values to their children. The behavior half of this is the most obvious and parents often use it as an indicator as to whether the values have been absorbed. This doesn't always work. In many families parents have effective control over much of the behavior of their young teens. They may control by strength, with no passage of any value but that of "might is right." When these teens grow older, out of their parents' control, they've learned few values but to resist their parents' overtures. They will not be open to further learning.

Parents will find it more effective to emphasize first the values behind behaviors, as Jesus did. After this emphasis, after parents' values have been firmly stated, then strength may be used to control young teens' behavior if parents feel this is essential. With young teens, the parents' control of their behavior is one effective way of parents' living and modeling their own values.

Fifteen year old Rick wants to go to an X-rated movie with the gang.

Rick: "Aw . . . but dad, it's not so bad. Some of the guys have gone before and they say there's nothin' to it."

Dad: "Rick, I feel that movies like that are degrading to both women and men. You know they make sex seem like something dirty. The actors must not value themselves very highly if they sell themselves for so little."

Rick: "But I promise, I'll mow the lawn every Saturday for you. I'll show you I'm old enough. All the guys are going. I'll be left out!"

Dad: "No, I won't sell my values. And this really has nothing to do with your age or how responsible you are. I don't want to separate you from your friends, but I feel very strongly about those movies. By paying to see them, you're supporting their false values. And I don't want you to grow up thinking sex is as they show it in those movies. So, you're just not going to go. We'll plan to do something else Friday evening."

Rick: "Aw, rats!"

Rick is not happy with this. But dad is firm. He can still control Rick's behavior. He doesn't criticize Rick or put down his friends or make deals. Dad sticks to just the central question and explains his values about it before laying down the ultimatum. Dad's primary goal is not to break the peer pressure on Rick, not to get Rick to be more responsible or have the lawn mowed regularly, so he passes over these unrelated and therefore minor issues, putting them in perspective. His real goal is to impart values about degrading sexuality and so this is what he centers his conversation on.

Conflicts with older teens have to be worked through a bit differently. Parents expect to lose direct control over their children's behavior around the seventeenth birthday. This varies, of course, according to whether the older teens are living at home or away at school, whether they use the family car and whether they depend upon the family or their own earnings for clothing or meals. Whatever the situation, parents would do well not to depend on strict control of behavior for solving conflicts or enforcing values. As these teens approach young adulthood, they need to "practice" being adults. This is not to say that parents should drop them like a lead balloon, but they should be supportive and continue to help their children's values and outlook on life toward maturity. At this age, teens are very sensitive to which values are actually successful in life. As parents lose control, or gradually relinquish it willingly, they must make extra efforts to model their own values to their older teens and young adult children. There are two phases to this modeling: a clear and mature statement of the parents' values; and parents' behavior, acting on these values, that show that the values really work in this world. Older teens are becoming more adept at consciously analyzing what they see around them. They will certainly reject values and attitudes that they perceive as bringing failure and unhappiness in adult life.

This situation causes the greatest challenge of all to parents. It calls into question the parents as successful persons. It puts them under examination and judgment by their offspring. It requires them to prove the successfulness of the values they've chosen to live their lives by. It is just this challenge that causes the worst dilemma for Catholic parents today. Are Catholic values successful in this world? What is success? By what standard are we judging? A genuine conflict with an older teen or young adult puts a parent on the knife-edge of life.

Nineteen year old Keith has brought his girl Cindy home from college for the weekend. They had intended to sleep together in Keith's room. The conversation has already covered the parents' disapproval of the proposed sleeping arrangements. That phase closed with the parents' firm statement about what they value as standards of behavior in their house. Keith has put forward, as one of his justifications, the fact that Cindy has been using a contraceptive pill. Keith seems to feel that this makes their sexual relationship all right, with no serious consequences. Mom and dad have kept the discussion on the conversational level. They are concerned that Keith and Cindy are very casual about their sexual relationship, and they want to keep the conversation going so that they might have some chance to influence them.

Mom: "Keith, I'm concerned about how you feel about using contraceptives."

Keith: "Yeah? It's a good thing to have. We wouldn't want Cindy to get pregnant. She has to finish school, and I need to graduate and get a job before we think about that."

Mom: "Well, I'm glad you're clear on the importance of your education. You seem to care enough about one another not to put an end to your plans in that way. But how do you feel about sex, then? What is the reason for it?"

Keith: "Huh?"

Dad: "She means, why have sex?"

Keith: "Because we love each other . . . it makes us feel great. Isn't that the way it's supposed to be?"

Dad: "Yes, it should bring you together, it should be great, but your mother and I believe there should be more to it than just that."

Keith: "More?"

Mom: "Keith, a sexual relationship is much more than just the time you spend in bed with each other. It's your whole life of commitment to each other. Your father and I feel that, for some people, the easy use of contraceptives can take away that deep commitment and make a relationship shallow and casual."

Keith: "Holy cow! I can't believe you'd want us to risk getting pregnant. And how come you have no children younger than Tommy? He's fourteen."

Dad: "Of course we don't want you to risk pregnancy. But we *do* want you to grow into an appreciation of the real value of a sexual relationship, not just as a way to feel good."

Mom: "You're right, Keith. Your father and I decided that we just couldn't have any more children after Tommy. That was when he was out of work, and we didn't know what the future would bring. Later, we felt we were just getting too old."

Dad: "Your mother and I use natural family planning, Keith. It's a way of controlling our family size while respecting what we feel is God's will for our sexuality. At first it wasn't easy. But it really means a lot to us now. You know, I think we love each other more now than we did then."

Keith: "But what does that have to do with me and Cindy?"

Mom: "We think your love might have more chance to grow and you'd be able to develop a deeper relationship if you took your sexual expression more seriously. We feel that your contraceptive use might be preventing this, that it makes sex easy and cheap and of little value."

Keith: "Naw . . . I don't know . . . it sounds too risky to me."

Dad: "Well, think about it while you're here, in separate bedrooms. And if you want to talk more later, we're here."

Keith's parents know that they can't force Keith and Cindy to change. A hellfire-and-brimstone sermon would only force them away from any future conversation or influence. Mom and dad have stuck to their own values on the bedroom arrangement. They have set forth their beliefs about contraceptive use and have allowed Keith to see how they've lived out their values. If it's obvious to Keith that they love one another, if they let him see some of their genuine affection and depth of relationship, then he will know that this strategy works in real life, not just in flashy brochures and well-written homilies. He may not change right away, but he's been given a solid foundation block; he's been set to thinking. He's been shown a facet of Christian life that is proven successful.

How can we show Christian values to be successful in our lives when they often cause us times of hardship and denial? Since the time of St. Paul, this task has been taken up, and sometimes done poorly, sometimes well. Here's one last example. Henry's dad has been divorced for five years. Henry is twenty and lives with his dad in their large house. Dad has dated several women over the years, but none have made him as happy as Ruth, whom he is seeing now. Henry likes her, too. They've spent the day cross-country skiing and the evening romantically curled up before a fire in the den while Henry worked on a term paper. Dad is now returning from driving Ruth home.

Henry: "Gee, dad, you're back awfully soon."

Dad: (laughs) "It's just three miles."

Henry: "Yeah, but I expected you to stay there a while at least, or maybe overnight."

Dad: "Oh no—no overnight."

Henry: "Why not, dad? You really love each other, don't you?"

Dad: "Yes, we do. That's why no overnight."

Henry: "Huh?"

Dad: "Love is very special to me, Henry. I know what it's like to have love and lose it, to be empty and lonely. Love was cheap and superficial for me once. I know better now."

Henry: "Yeah, but I mean, what about sex? If you love each other so much, you must want to have sex."

Dad: "Well, I guess we do. But, you know, we put a very high value on ourselves, and our sexual expression as well. We may want to get married."

Henry: "Great! But then there's no reason not to have sex. You were both married before, so it's not as though you're virgins or something like that."

Dad: "Henry, love is a commitment, and intercourse is one of the highest expressions of that commitment. We both know what it means to have a commitment fail. Ruth and I believe in marriage. We'll complete our commitment in love on the evening we complete our commitment to the community."

Henry: "But what if you find out then that you're not compatible?"

Dad: (laughing again) "Henry, your sexual expression is just that—an expression of who you are and how much you love, not the other way around. If we've found ourselves compatible in other things, then we'll be compatible sexually. What differences there are bound to be, we'll work on. That's what love means."

Henry: "Yeah, but . . ."

Dad: "I've got to go to bed now, kid. Why don't you go back to work on that paper, and we'll talk some more later."

Henry: "Yeah, but . . ."(Dad leaves.)

The Playboy philosophy notwithstanding, Henry sees his dad as a success. Dad does not mope, frown or express tension or impatience at waiting for sexual gratification until remarriage. He is happy with his choices and lets Henry know. Both are fully aware of the time of loneliness, but dad doesn't dwell on this now. He has chosen a course for life that works. He is not afraid to be transparent to his child. He doesn't need to give a theological background for his beliefs or quote Scripture. Those aren't his personal style. To let his son know his choice and see that his contentment with it is real—this is the example that teaches the value.

We've seen that the techniques involved in talking about sex with teens and young adults are basically an extension of those used with younger children. Add to these the teen's strong need for love, shown by parents in time, attention, and acceptance. Finally, add on the clear statement and genuine modeling of mature values, and we have the picture. Sometimes problems, conflicts, or crises develop that parents just cannot deal with. Then it is time to seek competent help from clergy, pastoral personnel, or professional counselors. Parents need not be hesitant or ashamed to turn for help. The tensions in our world are great, and none of us can be expected to cope alone with every possible situation.

The single most important step in talking about sex with anyone, young children, teens, or young adults, is simply to open one's mouth, to begin the process, to *talk*. Don't fear mistakes. They are unavoidable anyway, but be sure to correct the mistakes. Here's where the real learning happens. You don't need to be an expert biologist or psychologist or theologian, but to be open and willing to learn, to read a book or two, and to buy at least one good one the whole family can read. Tell the truth as simply as possible, fitting the explanation to the developmental level of the child. Learn to keep conversations going without the judgment and condemnation that will end them permanently. Check out what your child needs and wants with sincere and casual questions, not interrogations. Keep your own emotions under strict control; your background is much different, more complicated, than that of your children. They don't have in mind all the implications of their questions that you may. Don't lose sight of your real goals: to provide information, to instill values, to affect behaviors. Muddying sexual conversations with other issues will only draw you away from those goals. Spend time with your children, and during this time show your love with genuine and focused attention, talk, and enjoyment of their company.

Learn to know your own values clearly and live them so that your children can see that those values are successful. Tell your children, by your life, that Christian values really work. As your children grow through their teens into young adulthood, learn to let them go from your direct influence, but keep them coming back by talking and sharing your feelings and values. If they make choices you don't agree with, don't drive them away but help them live with them. They now have their own consciences, for which they are responsible. Keep the conversation open and model your life for them to cling to when they suffer failures.

By far, the best time to start talking to children about sexuality is in the months before they are born. But if you haven't started yet, it's still not too late. Whether you have infants, young children, preteens, teens, or young adults, you can begin where you are. Granted, it is more difficult the older the child. But it's never too late to absorb a loss, so start right now. Your children get older by the minute.

Typical Questions Children Ask

PRE-SCHOOL
1. How did the baby get in your tummy?
2. What's that (pointing to mom's breast)? Why is it bigger than mine?
3. How come I have a penis and you don't?
4. What is a rubber?
5. What's that, daddy? (daughter points to penis)
6. What's that, mommy? (son points to breasts)
7. How long does a baby grow inside its mother?
8. Where did I come from?
9. Does it hurt the mother to have a baby?
10. How did I get inside mama?
11. How are babies born?
12. Why don't I have one of those? (girl points to little boy's penis)
13. Why does my penis get hard?
14. What are these (tampons, sanitary napkins) for?
15. How did I eat inside you, mom?
16. Why do I have a belly button?
17. Why can't I have a penis?
18. What's down here between my legs? (for girls)
19. What's this little bump that feels good when I touch it? (clitoris)
20. Why can't I pee in the bath water?
21. Why can't I play with my urine?

22. Why is a BM dirty?
23. Why do I have to put clothes on?
24. Why do I have to go to the bathroom? I like to do it better outside.
25. Do you have to be married to have a baby?

ABOUT 6–9
1. How many ways can you get pregnant and what are the ways?
2. Does it hurt to have a baby?
3. Where does a baby come from?
4. How many times do people have to have intercourse to have a baby?
5. Why don't boys get breasts?
6. Do boys have anything like periods?
7. What are homosexuals?
8. How do you get twins?
9. What does menstruate mean?
10. What's a tampon? Sanitary pad?
11. Why don't girls like to play baseball?
12. How can I get a boy to like me?
13. Why can't we take baths together anymore?
14. How does the baby grow inside the mother?
15. Why do only mothers have babies?
16. How can a whole baby grow from only two cells?
17. How does a baby come out?
18. Why is it bad to say "fuck"?
19. Why can't I have a baby now?
20. What does "rape" mean?

ABOUT 10–13
1. How is sperm released into the female?
2. What are wet dreams?
3. Why do our bodies need to change?
4. What is masturbation? Is it harmful?
5. What's wrong with Playboy magazine or nude pictures?
6. Why do girls have periods?
7. Why is my penis smaller than yours? (son asks father)
8. Does it hurt to have sexual intercourse?
9. What does it mean to be queer? (homosexual)
10. What does "coming" mean?
11. Why do people have sexual intercourse?
12. Why don't boys have periods?
13. What are the first signs of pregnancy?

14. What is VD? (venereal disease)
15. Should you know how to do "it"?
16. How do you know when puberty is over?
17. Can a male release sperm without really knowing it?
18. At what age do you say a boy or girl should have sex?
19. Can urine come out at the same time sperm do?
20. When do you know when you're grown up?
21. Where does the milk come from in the breasts?
22. Why don't men make milk?
23. Does the penis have to be hot before it can give off sperm?
24. How often does the man give off sperm?
25. How do you come on to a girl to have sex?
26. Could a man have a disease in his sperm? Will it affect the baby?
27. How does a mother's skin stretch to let the baby grow?
28. Why do some people have miscarriages?
29. What is an abortion? How does it work?
30. If the mother is already pregnant and she has intercourse, what will happen?
31. If the baby is born dead, why did it die?
32. Why do some girls look fully grown at thirteen and some do not?
33. How come some girls can't have babies?
34. Why does it hurt the first time you have intercourse?
35. Does the penis have to be erect to have intercourse? If it isn't, does it hurt?
36. If you only have sex once, can you get pregnant?
37. If you have sex when you're young, can you or the baby die?
38. How should you act when you have your period?
39. Why does the baby grow faster in the uterus than outside?
40. What happens if a girl doesn't menstruate by the time she's sixteen?
41. How do babies get the milk out of the nipple?
42. When a baby develops, how does it become a girl or a boy?
43. How do doctors know when babies will be born?
44. Will it affect the baby if the mother or father drinks or takes drugs?
45. Is it a sin to have intercourse before you're married?
46. What are some ways to impress girls? (boys)

AGE 14 AND UP
1. What is the best birth control method?
2. Is love a good reason to have sex?
3. Do the sex organs stop operating after a certain age?
4. At what age do you think it is best to have children?
5. Does it hurt when a guy and you go all the way?
6. What should you do if you think you have VD?

7. What is masturbation? Is it harmful?
8. Is there any physical damage done by swallowing your sperm?
9. Is it wrong to masturbate with other people?
10. Do your nipples get hard when you get excited?
11. Do two people in love tend to separate from others?
12. Why do two people fall in love?
13. Can you have mature love at my age?
14. Can you like someone if your friend also likes him (her)?
15. When do you tell a guy to stop? How far do you let him go?
16. What is a French kiss? Is it a sin?
17. If you like someone, how do you tell him (her)?
18. What is the age that people may start a good relationship?
19. What is immature love?
20. If you're really in love, is it okay to have sex before marriage?
21. How do you act when you are around a guy and you're shy?
22. How can I make boys (girls) like me?
23. How can I tell if someone is really in love with me and not just saying so?

Questions for Discussion

1. Why does talking about sexual matters tend to be very difficult for many adults today? What is the history of this?
2. What are the normal first communications about sexuality with young children? How can these be positive or negative?
3. Why is learning to ask your children questions important? What would be a helpful way to ask a question? What would be a harmful way?
4. What is the one greatest commandment of talking to children about sex? How does this work?
5. Why is the fear of making mistakes important? What can parents do if they've made a mistake when talking about sex with their children?
6. How do you deal with sexual slang in your home? Are there some words that make you personally upset? How can you learn to cope with these? Do you feel somewhat insensitive to sexual slang? What can you do about this?
7. Why is time spent with their parents important to teenagers? How can parents provide this time?
8. Why must teens and young adults be able to see their parents' values as successful? How can parents insure that this will happen?
9. Why is the "big talk" approach not effective sexuality education? How, then, can parents be sure that all important areas of knowledge are discussed with their children?
10. How can some of the principles of everyday sexual conversations be put into practice in conflict situations? What additional guidelines would be helpful?

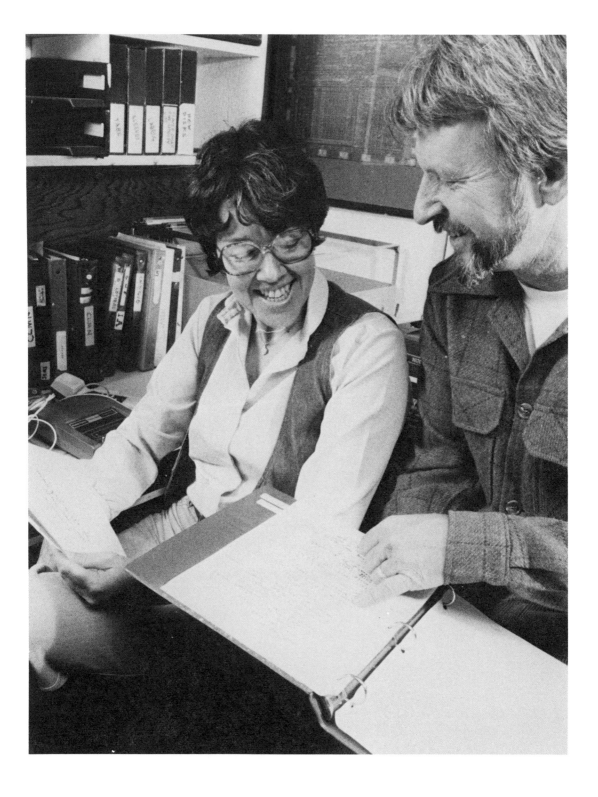

Resources for Parents
or
Where Do We Go from Here?

Throughout this book we have acknowledged our limitations and urged parents to seek out additional sources of information and support. We have tried to provide a unique blend of explanation and encouragement. This book is simply an overview to help you realize that the task of raising children to be sexually and spiritually healthy and secure is infinitely important and not beyond your ability. But neither is it easy. Parents need all the support they can get. You will most certainly need to look further than this book as questions, situations, and problems arise in your family life. This is to be expected. But where can you turn?

Many services and resources are available. The trick lies in choosing those that will be most helpful to you. Some of these are Catholic in origin and values; some are not specifically Catholic, but still Christian in outlook; vastly more are secular, or non-value oriented or "value free." When faced with this range of possibilities, many people feel overwhelmed, confused, or threatened.

The first source of support most people turn to is quite naturally other people, friends, neighbors, other family members, or even parents. Most of our life-knowledge continues to be passed on this way. This is probably good. But just a word of caution. We have seen that very often sexual untruths, myths, or downright misinformation is passed along in this way. It is hard to sort out the valuable, common wisdom from the incorrect information or unhealthy attitudes. As comforting as grandma's old sayings or the consensus of the coffee klatch may be, as well meaning as best friends are, often something more is needed.

The next direction most people turn in search of help and guidance may be their Church. The Church's traditional role of teacher reinforces this tendency. But the Church's history of a simplistic rather than holistic approach to teaching about sexuality and family life may also cause some people to hold back, unwilling to approach when they believe there is no real help available. Quotes from papal statements taken out of context and turned to the media's usual style of sensationalism give a false impression of the Church's teaching and attitudes about sexuality today. Occasional unfortunate homilies by overworked, understaffed, undertrained, and aging pastors can reinforce people's negative feelings about the Church and sexuality. In previous chapters, we have tried to explain how some traditional beliefs about the relationship between spirituality and sexuality came about. They evolved gradually, over time. They were added to or modified often as new theologians or traditions influenced the Church. But most people don't stop to realize that this process is still going on. As new medical knowledge is available and as theologians continue to study and wrestle with questions of sexuality, the Church continues to change. Admittedly, this change is subtle and slow. But it is happening nevertheless.

Vatican Council II gave this change a tremendous boost in many areas. One of the most significant is the shift in emphasis of Church teaching from an act-centered and rather legalistic morality, to a person-centered point of view. With this in mind we can begin to expect more genuine guidance from the Church in leading our personal lives.

But, again, the Church is very large. This means that growth and change are slow. We need both patience and persistence when we turn to the Church for help and resources in sexuality-related matters. The first aspect of the Church available to people is their parish priest. We must not be willing to give in to frustration if the first parish priest we meet does not particularly have the talent, personality, or specialized training to deal with sexuality-related questions or problems. The Church needs a vast variety of talents. Few men can or should try to fill all the needs of all the people. Just as some are better liturgists, or more adept at administration, some priests are more comfortable interpreting the Church's guidance in sexual matters. It is up to you to search out these pastoral people when you need them. They are living and working in every diocese. Word of mouth from other parishioners or perhaps a diocesan referral service can put you in touch with them.

The next Church-related function parents should consider looking into is their own Diocesan Family Life or Human Development Office. Though the names vary from one diocese to another, most have some centralized agency that develops, coordinates, or offers programs to enrich family and personal life. These services may include pre-Cana workshops, divorced and separated groups, family planning classes and seminars, pro-life and other consciousness-raising and lobbying groups, family enrichment workshops, family retreat programs, homes for battered women, services for pregnant teens, soup kitchens, and housing services, ethnic and bilingual programs, and many, many more. Hopefully your diocese will have some program that deals with your particular needs. If not, they should be able to refer you to a priest-counselor or private counselor who can give you individual guidance.

In many areas, where towns are far distant from diocesan centers or services, secular services and resources may be most obvious, most convenient, and least expensive. They are often funded by government or private grants, community charities, or directly by tax dollars. Their staff are usually well-trained professionals. Their printed materials are well-planned, attractive and readable. In many communities they may seem to be the only resource, and in some they are. It is important that parents become mature and secure enough in their faith to be able to deal with these secular resources. Jesus' example shows us that we should not withdraw from the world, but rather live in it and work to convert it around ourselves. We cannot isolate ourselves out of fear or try to become an exclusive community. The test of our faith comes in our ability to find what is good and useful within secular resources, to decide what is right for ourselves and reject what is not a part of our value structure. As Catholics we are called by the Spirit to bring the world to Christ by example, not by isolation.

If, in conscience, you cannot deal with a particular agency because of their differing value structure or stand on a particular issue, then by all means do not hesitate to look elsewhere for education and services. If you find yourself involved with a particular service group and you become uncomfortable with their advice or practices, then you need not feel tied down. Just as every good doctor will not fear a second opinion, neither should an individual or group working in the realm of sexuality become offended if some people would prefer not to use their services.

These are some of the kinds of services you may be able to find in your community: child birth classes, child rearing and nutritional information, parenting workshops, support groups for single parents, pregnancy testing services, VD clinics, rape crisis services, medical hotline, adoption services, parent-child and couple communication workshops, divorced, separated and widowed groups, support groups and homes for pregnant teens, counseling services for families, adults, teens, educational resource centers which provide films, speakers, pamphlets and books, continuing education courses at high schools and colleges, and more.

Another resource which certainly has value is books. We are often told, "But parents don't have time to read." That may be true, but you have to do something after the kids have gone to bed, and you're too exhausted to do any more work. Turn off the boob tube once a week and spend an evening munching popcorn and reading a good book about sex. If we work hard enough, we may make it sound almost as appealing as the "soaps." Well . . . almost. The truth is, reading a good book about sex is cheaper, probably more interesting, and certainly more productive than ninety percent of today's TV shows. But again, as with community services, we have the old problem of fear. "What if the book says something that isn't right?" Medically, scientifically, and statistically, most books published in the last five to ten years are probably pretty close to correct. Look for well-known publishing companies and fairly recent copyright dates. In matters of faith and morals, look for the

"Imprimatur" on the same page as the publishing information. This is the Church's official statement that the content is free of errors in faith or moral teaching. After these two guides, you are again on your own regarding the opinions and values presented in a book. Some books containing sexuality-values material are quite "liberal"; some are "conservative" or even "reactionary." You have to use your own God-given mind and powers of judgment. Remembering the values you have absorbed throughout your life, from your own parents, from experience, and from the guiding Church, judge the book by its contents, not by the cover, the reputation of the author, or the most vocal of your circle of friends. If you find yourself holding a book which offends you, put it down. No one learns when being offended. Don't feel you have to make yourself uncomfortable. Often both the over-conservative and the over-liberal critics will blast a particular book for completely opposite reasons. That's probably the book you'll enjoy reading the most. Be selective with books just as you would be with services.

Where can one find good books on sexuality? In many unlikely places. We were once criticized for recommending the library as a service. Evidently the critic felt that the library was full of secular, value-free books that would certainly be harmful. A mature and thoughtful person can make decisions about library books on the individual merits of each. Library books are inexpensive, varied in reading level, interest level, and specific content areas. If you want a book on the biology of the reproductive systems, you can get just that, or one on papal statements or Church teaching or secular humanism. Librarians can help look up specific topics in books or in periodicals and guide you to current periodicals and literature on sexuality, Church, and other issues. Quite a few editions and translations of the Bible are even found in most libraries.

Many bookstores now have specific sections devoted to sexuality, family studies, women's issues, or health. Occasionally these books will be limited to the more sensational and less educational varieties of sexual books. But most bookstores will order for you any books they don't normally stock if you know the name of the book you want. Very good books are sometimes found in supermarkets, drugstores, and department stores. Religious bookstores are another source and they can also order books for you. If you are still a bit timid, or don't even know quite what you want, ask your priest or pastoral person to help you in selecting what would be just right for you.

It is important that we think a bit now about books and children. Books can be an excellent resource in teaching your children about their sexuality. But if you bring books into your home for this purpose, you should be sure to read them carefully yourself first. First of all, you want to be as knowledgeable as your children. It's silly to try to teach them something you don't know yourself. Second, you want to be prepared to discuss any issues or questions that arise from reading a particular book. Many books will be entirely acceptable, but there may be one or two specific points that you may wish to review and clarify with your children. In the case of young children, you may need to check the vocabulary to see that they will be able to understand it. They may need parts read to them. Older children who have not had a chance to really talk about sexuality before, may prefer to read on their own at first before opening up to conversations about sex.

At the end of this chapter, you will find a bibliography of books concerning various aspects of sexuality. These are by no means all of the books that exist in this topic area. We are constantly adding to our list as new books come to our attention. Not all of these books will be appropriate for every reader. We offer you this list with the requirement that you be mature in your judgment and choices. We expect you to take responsibility for what you read and bring into your home. Your backgrounds, tastes and opinions are all different. We expect you to let others be different from you. We have tried to include books that will be helpful to as many different parents and children as possible.

Just a final word of encouragement: be confident in your striving for growth in your sexual knowledge. Ignorance is never bliss. It is an uneasy peace at best, and an open door to exploitation and tragedy at worst. Jesus never meant truth or knowledge or wisdom or understanding to be withheld from anyone. With the help of the Spirit, we should make efforts to learn what is necessary for a well-adjusted and positive family life.

Questions for Discussion

1. Make a list of the services available to you through the Church in your own diocese.
2. Make a list of the services available to you in your secular community.
3. Which secular services would you prefer not to use and why? Which could you benefit from the most?
4. Is there some need that is not being fulfilled by your Church, nor in a form that you can make use of in your community? Whom in your diocesan office could you call about developing a program to fill this need?
5. What are some of the benefits and dangers of turning to friends and relatives when information and wisdom about sexual matters is needed?
6. Why have people tended not to turn to the Church for help in sexually-related matters in the recent past?
7. Why do some people fear community agencies that deal with sexual resources? Is this fear well-founded? How could someone overcome this hesitancy and use a resource that is needed?
8. Why are there such a variety of books on sexuality, and how would you go about selecting one for your family?
9. What books on sexuality have you already read and found helpful? If you haven't, what particular kind of book are you interested in reading first?

Other Family Reading About Sexuality

We believe that it is helpful to read about sexuality from a variety of sources. Every author phrases things differently, and opinions may vary, but established facts do not, and from such differences comes the responsibility to learn to make one's own choices and decisions based on our values, beliefs, and facts.

The books on the following reading list have been selected for different ages and different special needs. Many have been recommended to us. We have read some, but unfortunately, because of the time involved, we have not been able to read and screen them all. This list will be useful not only for parents and young people, but also for teachers, counselors, clergy and youth leaders.

One of the best ways to encourage open communication about sexuality with your family is to have several books on the subject for various ages around the house, easily accessible to everyone. Since individuals of the same age vary greatly in maturity, it is important for a family bookshelf to include a wide variety to cover the needs of different age groups. It is also recommended that parents be familiar with a book before they share it with their children, but they should always remember that no matter how good the book, it can never replace a parent willing and able to talk about sex with a child.

YOUNG CHILDREN AND THEIR PARENTS

How Babies Are Made by Andrew C. Andry and Steven Shepp. The story of reproduction in plants, animals and humans, told through color photographs of paper sculptures. Factually accurate and easily understood.
(New York: Time-Life Inc., 1968)

Did the Sun Shine Before You Were Born? by S. Gordon and Gordon. A book which parents can read with their children ages 3–6. In addition to answering the question "Where do babies come from?" clearly and directly, it deals with other aspects of how different kinds of families live and grow.
(New York: Ed-U Press, 1977)

Growing Up Feeling Good: A Child's Introduction to Sexuality by Stephanie Waxman. An excellent introduction to many important concepts about human sexuality, presented with simplicity and dignity.
(California: Panjandium Books, 1979)

Our New Baby: A Picture Story About Birth for Parents and Children by Grethe Fagerstrom and Gunilla Hansson. Story of a year a new baby arrives, and the parents and children discuss how she was conceived, developed and born, and what she means to the family.
(New York: Barron's Educational Series, 1982)

How Was I Born? A Photographic Story of Reproduction and Birth for Children by Lennart Nilsson. Tells the story of reproduction and birth using the famous Nilsson photographs of fetal development with warm family scenes and other illustrations.
(New York: Delacorte Press, 1975)

The Wonderful Story of How You Were Born by Sidonie Matsner Gruenberg. Explains for young children how life begins and develops from the union of a sperm and an egg. Human and animal parents are contrasted and the changes in a new baby's body as it matures are described. This book is now a classic.
(New York: Doubleday and Co., Inc., 1973)

What Is a Girl? What Is a Boy? by Stephanie Waxman. A simply written, non-sexist message for young children: names, hair lengths, interests, clothing, and emotions do not identify a person as a boy or a girl—only a person's genitals can do that.
(Culver City, CA: Peace Press, 1976)

Learning About Sex by Jennifer J. Aho and J.W. Petras. Helpful for parents to use with children. Includes beautiful illustrations.
(New York: Holt, Rinehart and Winston, 1978)

Where Do Babies Come From?: by Margaret Sheffield. Very simple and complete explanations of intercourse, pregnancy and birth.
(New York: Alfred A. Knopf, 1973)

Let's Find Out About Babies by M. Shapp, C. Shapp, and S. Shepard. Very good to read to young children; basic idea that babies come from loving parents and are like them.
(New York: Franklin Watts, Inc., 1974)

A Baby Starts To Grow by Paul Shawere. Can be read to young children, good illustrations, accurate and simple wording of growth of baby.
(New York: Thomas Y. Crowell Co., 1969)

PRE-TEENS AND THEIR PARENTS

Love and Sex and Growing Up by Corinne Benson Johnson and Eric W. Johnson. Deals with many topics to help elementary-age children think about being a man or a woman and what this means.
(New York: Bantam Books Inc., 1979)

Period by JoAnn Gardner-Loulan, Bonnie Lopez and Marcia Quackenbush. Reassuring, cleverly illustrated book about menstruation. Explains why all girls are normal, yet each one is special. Includes personal narratives.
(San Francisco: Volcano Press, 1979)

Girls' Guide to Menstruation by Ellen Vaelechers. Excellent, thorough explanation of menstruation, hygiene and health; good pictures and diagrams, easy to read.
(New York: Richard Rosen Press, Inc., 1975)

The Human Story, Facts on Birth, Growth and Reproduction by Sadie Hofstein. Clear description of reproduction for reference or to be read by pre-teens.
(Dallas, TX: Scott, Foresman and Co., 1977)

EARLY TEENS AND THEIR PARENTS

Love and Sex in Plain Language by Eric W. Johnson. Basic information on sexuality, emphasizing that it should always be seen in the context of one's total personality and expressed in responsible, respectful caring relationships.
(Paper: New York: Bantam Books, Inc., 1979)

Learning About Sex: The Contemporary Guide for Young Adults by Gary F. Kelly. This book, while giving basic factual information, focuses on attitudes and the process of making sexual decisions responsibly.
(Woodbury, NY: Barron's Educational Series Inc., 1977)

Are You There, God? It's Me, Margaret by Judy Blume. Reassuring story about pre-adolescent girls as they face the physical changes that usually accompany puberty as well as peer pressure.
(New York: Yearling Books, Dell, 1974)

Forever by Judy Blume. Its reception by adolescents has made this book a classic. A story of first love with explicit passages about the adolescents' sexual experiences.
(Paper: New York: Pocket Books, 1975)

Sex, Sexuality and You: A Handbook for Growing Christians by Nancy Hennessy Cooney. Provides accurate sexual information in the context of a Catholic value system.
(Dubuque, Iowa: William C. Brown Co., 1980)

Boys and Sex, Girls and Sex by Wardell B. Pomeroy. Sexual guides for boys and girls written in straightforward, objective, and non-judgmental ways, using language which is easily understood.
(New York: Delacorte Press, 1981, revised edition)

Sex with Love: A Guide for Young People by Eleanor Hamilton. Complete guide to the young person who needs to reflect on decisions about sexual activity.
(Boston: Beacon Press, 1978)

Preparing for Adolescence by James Dobson. Written in clear, direct langauge which gives facts about menstruation, masturbation, venereal disease and other topics.
(Santa Ana, CA: Vision House Publishers, 1978)

Sexuality and Dating: A Christian Perspective by Richard Reichert. Offers young people a clear and integrated discussion of their own sexual development and of the present challenges in achieving sexual and moral maturity as Christians.
(Winona, MN: St. Mary's Press, 1981)

LATER TEENS AND THEIR PARENTS

Sex and Birth Control: A Guide for the Young, Revised Edition by James Lieberman and Ellen Peck. Direct and honest presentation for young people that encourages them to develop principles and values by which they will live their sexual lives.
(New York: Harper and Row, 1981)

What's the Matter with Me? by Eda LeShan. Excellent discussion for young people on the problems of the teen years; easy to read.
(New York: Scholastic Book Services, 1974)

Commonsense Sex by Ronald M. Mazur. Based on the premise that sex is a positive aspect of human personality and concludes with a suggestion of a liberal religious framework for decision making.
(Boston: Beacon Press, 1968)

The Facts of Love: Living, Loving and Growing Up by Alex Comfort and Jane Comfort. A dynamic book about sexuality; ideal as a catalyst for conversations with young people.
(New York: Ballantine Books, 1980, paperback edition)

ESPECIALLY FOR PARENTS

Sex: The Facts, The Acts, and Your Feelings by Michael Carrera. Comprehensive, in-depth, easy to understand information about sexuality, presented in a non-judgmental tone, but imparting values concerning people and relationships.
(New York: Crown Publishers, 1981)

Parenting: A Guide for Young People by S. Gordon and Mina Wallin. Practical guide for young adults needing helpful information on parenthood.
(New York: Sadlier-Oxford, 1983)

The Family Book About Sexuality by Mary Calderone and Eric W. Johnson. A comprehensive approach to the family's understanding of the sexuality and sexual concerns of all its members.
(Paper: New York: Bantam Books, Inc., 1983)

On Becoming a Family: The Growth of Attachment by T. Berry Brazelton. In this wonderful book for all parents, and especially for parents to be, a well-known pediatrician reveals how the bonds between parents and baby are developed and deepened.
(Paper: New York: Dell Publishing Co., Inc., 1981)

Your Child and Sex: A Guide for Parents by Wardell B. Pomeroy. Gives parents a better understanding of their own sexuality, both in their marriage relationship and in their relationships with their children. Also deals with ways of talking about sex to children at various age levels from the very young to the post-adolescent.
(New York: Delacorte Press, 1974)

Talking with Your Child About Sex: Questions and Answers for Children from Birth to Puberty by Mary S. Calderone and James W. Ramey. Divided in six developmental sections from birth through age twelve. Each contains an introduction on that developmental stage, information about what to expect and how to deal with problems that might arise, and examples of questions children might ask about sex and samples of answers parents might give.
(New York: Random House, 1982)

Sex Without Shame: Encouraging the Child's Healthy Sexual Development by Alayne Yates. Explains primary facts about how children's sexuality develops and what parents can do to help.
(New York: William Morrow and Co., Inc., 1978)

Sex and the Single Parent by Jane Adams. Realistic portrait of intellectual and emotional struggles of single parents. Recommended for members of single parent families themselves, including adolescents.
(New York: Coward, McCann and Geoghegan, 1978)

Learning About Sex—A Guide for Children and Their Parents by Jennifer Aho and John Petras. Intended for parents to read with their children. A liberal attitude toward sex is projected, with emphasis on feelings and, especially, love. Discussion includes puberty, masturbation, pregnancy, birth, venereal disease, birth control. Beautiful illustrations accompany the discussions.
(New York: Holt, Rinehart, and Winston, 1978)

What To Say After You Clear Your Throat: A Parent's Guide to Sex Education by Jean S. Gochros. Discusses the art of communicating about sex with young people at various age levels. A special section on sex education and the handicapped is included.
(Hawaii: Press Pacifica, 1980)

Sex and the American Teenager by Murray M. Kappelman. Excellent work on how parents can better understand and help their teens to grow in responsible sexuality.
(New York: Readers Digest Press, 1977)

Sex and Your Teenager by Eda LeShan. Excellent work for parents of young people and later

teens; easy to read, with many examples.
(New York: David McKay Co., Inc., 1969)

A Family Guide to Sex by Isadore Rubin and Deryck Calderwood. Includes how to deal with pornography and obscenity, and what parents should know about homosexuality. Emphasizes that sex education belongs in the home.
(New York: New American Library, 1973)

When Children Ask About Sex: A Guide for Parents by Joan Selzer. Parents are provided with information about developmental issues. Emphasizes the positive aspects of loving, sex and marriage.
(Boston: Beacon Press, 1974)

Sex Education for Today's Child: A Guide for Modern Parents by Arlene S. Uslander, Caroline Weiss, and Judith Telman. Provides model answers to typical questions asked by children concerning sex.
(New York: Association Press, 1977)

Celebration in the Bedroom by Charlie Shedd and Martha Shedd. Explores the many ways in which it is possible to celebrate the gift of sexuality. Focuses on sexual enrichment for married couples who have made a commitment of fidelity to each other.
(Waco, TX: Word Books, 1979)

SPECIAL SUBJECTS

A Disturbed Peace: Selected Writings of an Irish-Catholic Homosexual by Brian McNaught. Serves as an excellent introduction to homosexuality for heterosexual people.
(Washington, DC: Dignity, Inc., 1981)

Raising a Child Conservatively in a Sexually Permissive World by S. Gordon and J. Gordon.
(New York: Simon and Schuster, 1983)

Psychology for You by S. Gordon. Excellent introductory course for high school students that applies psychology to personal problems and deals with a wide variety of social relationships.
(New York: Sadlier-Oxford, 1983)

Now That You Know: What Every Parent Should Know About Homosexuality by Betty Fairchild and Nancy Hayward. Informative, sensitively written guide for parents of homosexual children, but equally helpful for all parents whose children will eventually want to understand homosexual friends.
(Paper: New York: Harcourt Brace Jovanovich, 1981)

VD—And What You Should Do About It by Eric W. Johnson. For our age: facts simply given.
(New York: Harper and Row Inc., 1978)

The Silent Children—A Book for Parents About Prevention of Child Sexual Abuse by Linda Tschirhart Sanford. Deals with what families can do to prevent sexual abuse.
(New York: Anchor/Doubleday, 1980)

A Family Matter: A Parent's Guide to Homosexuality by Charles Silverstein. Written for parents of a homosexual child, this book examines the realities of the situation, and sug-

gests how to turn the experience into a positive relationship.
(New York: McGraw-Hill Book Co., 1977)

Growing Up Free: Raising Your Child in the '80s by Letty Cottin Pogrebin. Child-rearing from conception to puberty, emphasizing non-sexist education, parenting and gender-neutral attitude.
(Paper: New York: Bantam Books, Inc., 1981)

SEXUALITY AND RELIGION

What Are They Saying About Sexual Morality? by James Hanigan. Concise, readable and useful guide to recent developments in Catholic understanding about sexuality.
(Ramsey, New Jersey: Paulist Press, 1982)

And They Felt No Shame: Christians Reclaim Their Sexuality by Joan Ohanneson. Exciting, extensive knowledge of young adults (ages 18–35) and their search for affirmation that sex and sexuality are gifts from God to be enjoyed. Deals with issues in the Catholic tradition and challenges people of faith with a new understanding of sexuality.
(Minneapolis, MN: Winston Press, 1983)

The Good News About Sex by David Knight. For teens, the engaged, married couples, singles, parents, teachers, and clergy. Offers a positive view of sexuality. Challenges individuals towards high ideals in meaning and values.
(Cincinnati, Ohio: St. Anthony Messenger Press, 1979)

When It's Time To Talk About Sex by Gordon J. Lester. Focuses on a need to communicate reverence for sex, facilitates discovering sexual values and provides insights into mystery which reflects the life of God.
(St. Meinrad, Indiana: Abbey Press, 1981)

Patterns in Moral Development by Catherine M. Storehouse. Guidebook for parents and teachers facilitating the Christian moral development of children, youth and adults.
(Waco, TX: Word Incorporated, 1980)

A Parent's Guide to Sex and the Young Catholic by Gregory Kenny. Presents a clear, readable presentation of the Catholic understanding of sexuality for young people.
(Chicago: Claretian Publications, 1978)

The Church and the Homosexual by John J. McNeill. Extensive pastoral study of the moral concerns of homosexuality within the Catholic tradition.
(Kansas City: Sheed Andrews and McMeel, Inc., 1976)

Embodiment: An Approach to Sexuality and Christian Thinking by James B. Nelson. Significant dialogue on the theological meaning of human sexuality in the Christian community.
(Minneapolis: Augsburg Publishing House, 1978)

Homosexuality and Ethics by Edward Batchelor, Jr. ed. Selection of essays covering spectrum of Jewish, Protestant and Roman Catholic views on homosexuality.
(New York: Pilgrim Press, 1980)